ACUPRESSURE TAPING

The Practice of Acutaping for Chronic Pain and Injuries

Hans-Ulrich Hecker, M.D., and Kay Liebchen, M.D.

Translated from the German by Katja Lueders and Rafael Lorenzo

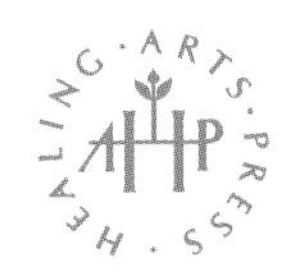

Healing Arts Press
Rochester, Vermont

Healing Arts Press
One Park Street
Rochester, Vermont 05767
www.HealingArtsPress.com

Healing Arts Press is a division of Inner Traditions International

Originally published in German under the title *Aku-Taping—sanft gegen den Schmerz* by Karl F. Haug Verlag in MVS Medizinverlage Stuttgart GmbH & Co. KG, Oswald-Hesse Straße 50 • 70469 Stuttgart, Germany
First U.S. edition published in 2007 by Healing Arts Press

Note to the reader: *This book is intended as an informational guide. The remedies, approaches, and techniques described herein are meant to supplement, and not to be a substitute for, professional medical care or treatment. They should not be used to treat a serious ailment without prior consultation with a qualified health care professional.*

Library of Congress Cataloging-in-Publication Data
[Aku-Taping. English]
Acupressure taping : the practice of acutaping for chronic pain and injuries / Hans-Ulrich Hecker and Kay Liebchen ; translated from the German by Katja Lueders and Rafael Lorenzo.
p. cm.
Includes index.
ISBN-13: 978-1-59477-148-4 (pbk.)
ISBN-10: 1-59477-148-0 (pbk.)
1. Acutaping—Popular works. 2. Chronic pain—Alternative treatment—Popular works. I. Liebchen, Kay. II. Title.
RM723.A28 2007
615.8'92—dc22

2006036739

Printed and bound in the United States by Versa Press, Inc.

10 9 8 7 6

Text design and layout by Priscilla Baker
This book was typeset in Sabon, with Avant Garde and Agenda used as display typefaces

Illustrations on pages 38–40 are from Schünke, Schulte, Schumacher, Voll, and Wesker, *Prometheus Allgemeine Anatomie und Bewegungssystem* (Stuttgart: Georg Thieme Verlag, 2004).

Interior taping photographs by Axel Nickolaus; all other photographs from the archives of Thieme Verlagsgruppe.

Contents

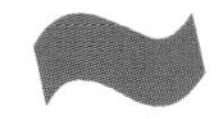

PART 2: HOW TO USE ACUTAPE 43

Introduction

Acutaping, if done properly, is a holistic and gentle approach to pain relief. As both a therapy and an approach to prevention, it is a helpful treatment for all sorts of chronic (recurring) and acute (severe) forms of pain.

This book is for people who are concerned with the issue of pain. It is also for people who are suffering from conditions that involve pain and for the therapists who treat them. We would like to present in this book a recently developed therapeutic method that can be used in a wide range of contexts—acutaping. In every situation, acutaping will show itself to be, as we state, "a gentle and holistic approach to pain relief."

In fact, the method described in this book makes it possible for people suffering from pain to ease or heal the pain by themselves. Moreover, a doctor or a therapist (massage therapist, physical therapist, chiropractor) can use this form of pain treatment as a way of actively involving the patient in the therapy. Thus, this book can be used as a guide both for self-treatment and for the practical cooperation of therapist and patient in the treatment process.

However, this book about acutaping cannot and should not replace a doctor's care. It is very important, as with any therapy, that a qualified physician looks into the cause of the pain. We would like to make this clear from the very start because we care for your well-being and the improper use of acutaping can do harm.

Pain can be divided into acute and chronic pain. Acute pain in a moving part of the body can be caused by a brief strain or a trauma, such as a sprained ankle or pulled muscle. Chronic pain for the most part is the result of a lingering strain or injury combined with a changing perception of pain and the movement of the pain to different parts of the body.

Pain reveals that there is a health problem—it does not matter if the pain is acute or if it is chronic. It is a signal from the body that should make a person conscious of a disturbance in the normally self-regulating procedures that ensure health. Thus, it is actually a positive sign in many respects.

Important!

No self-treatment without a doctor's diagnosis!

Functional problems can be caused by an underlying structural dysfunction. This is the reason why self-treatment can be dangerous without first getting a preliminary diagnosis from a doctor. Not seeking a doctor's help can lead to a dangerous delay in the detection of an underlying illness that might be the reason for the functional problem in the first place. So for any treatment with acutaping there is one hard-and-fast rule: any self-treatment with acutaping must be based on a doctor's diagnosis.

A health problem can be caused by either a functional or a structural disorder.

Examples of structural dysfunctions are a very bad abrasion of a joint, rheumatism, or a tumor. Yet these structural indispositions very often start with a functional and usually treatable illness that affects the way a part of the body works.

Besides using acutaping to treat acute and chronic pain, other ailments—such as internal or gynecological ones as well as sports injuries—also can be treated with acutaping. A recently developed method emphasizes preventive treatment for athletes—as well as for anyone else who is very active in sports. Here, acutaping is a prophylactic therapy, a preventive measure; and it has been used for such problem areas as the shoulder, knee, and ankle.

The tapes that we are introducing in the book are used in direct alignment with the part of the body that hurts. The description as to how the tapes are to be attached is based on knowledge gleaned from medical research.

Even someone with no experience of acupuncture can use the tapes. The taping is very easy, and the step-by-step process is thoroughly explained in the book. If you follow our directions, it will not be hard for you to attach the tapes. Your taping partner (the person who assists you in the taping) will find that this therapy really helps—and that taping is a lot of fun.

Important!

Find an acutaping partner!

Naturally, you need someone to help you attach the tapes in hard-to-reach or impossible-to-reach places such as the back. In fact, every taping requires a preliminary stretching movement in order to hold a posture while the tapes are applied, so you cannot attach the tape properly by yourself, anyway.

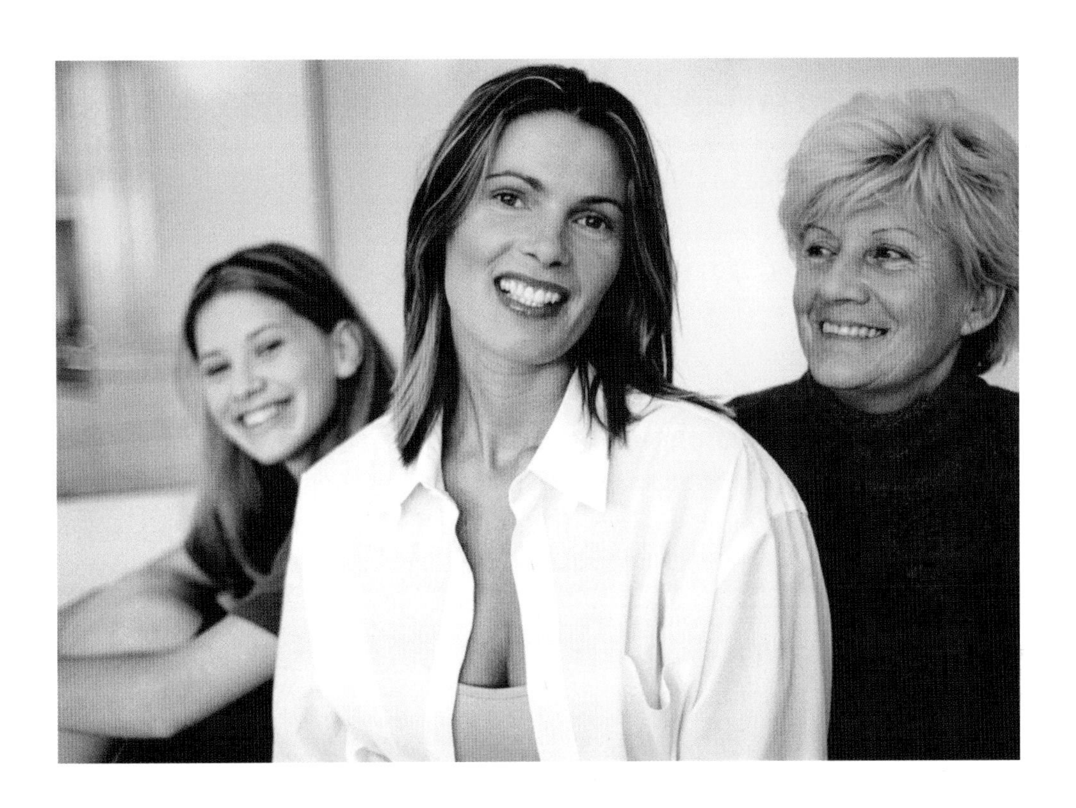

Part 1

WHAT IS ACUTAPING?

Acutaping is a relatively new therapy used in the treatment of pain that was developed by Hans-Ulrich Hecker, M.D., and Kay Liebchen, M.D. This method is based on kinesio-taping (a therapeutic technique in which elastic cotton tape is attached to the immediate area of a painful muscle, ligament, or joint) but also uses the diagnostic and therapeutic principles found in Chinese medicine, acupuncture, and acupressure.

What makes kinesio-taping unique is the nature of the tape itself. In contrast with conventional medicine, which uses tape as nonelastic, restrictive bandages for the purpose of binding and immobilizing joints, kinesio-tape bandages are, in fact, elastic and they support and encourage movement. It is this sort of elastic tape bandage that is used in acutaping as well.

Acutaping: A New Therapeutic Method

Acutaping is a new therapeutic method that uses flexible tape bandages on the basis of the theory of acupuncture.

The word *acutaping* combines the prefix "acu-" from the words *acupuncture* and *acupressure* with the word *tape*. An acupressure massage therapist uses finger pressure on the same points in which an acupuncturist inserts needles. In acutaping, the elastic tape often stimulates acupuncture/acupressure points related to the area where the patient feels pain. The term *acutaping* thus indicates that this is a new therapeutic method that establishes a connection between the theory of acupuncture/acupressure and the practice of kinesio-taping.

The difference between kinesio-taping and acutaping can be explained in this fashion: In kinesio-taping, the tapes are attached to the immediate area of a muscle, ligament, or joint that is in pain. In acutaping, along with these specific anatomical aspects at the locus of pain, the diagnostic and therapeutic rules of traditional Chinese medicine and acupuncture, as well as the manual medical approach of osteopathy, also are taken into consideration when placing the tapes. When these holistic methods of understanding are applied to the tape placements, the specific areas of the body that are taped may not necessarily be perceived as problem areas by the patient, yet tensions or blocked energy in these areas may be considered to have, in fact, an important causal relationship to the disorders or pain actually felt in other parts of the body.

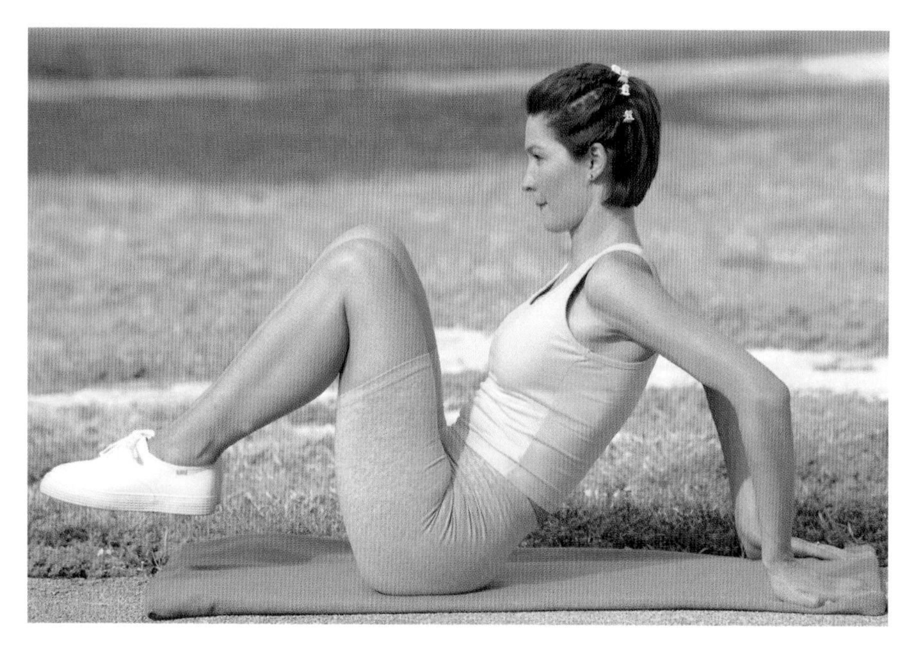

Unlike conventional medicine, which uses tape as nonelastic, restrictive bandages for the purpose of binding and immobilizing joints, acutaping does not inhibit freedom of movement.

The Foundation: Kinesio-Taping

In the early seventies, Japanese doctor and chiropractor Kenzo Kase developed kinesio-taping, which involves the use of elastic tape bandages along with other standard therapy methods. The tape itself is usually elastic along its length with some flexibility crosswise, and it conventionally is applied to the skin in the area of muscles and joints as they are held taut. As the muscle or joint moves, the tape bandage remains attached to the skin. In this way, there is a displacement of the skin against the tissue beneath the skin that creates an agitation of the muscle, ligament, or joint elements. In contrast with conventional nonelastic medical taping that is intended to keep the area immobile, flexible kinesio-tape actually supports and helps movement.

Kinesio-taping is effective in the treatment of disorders and dysfunctions of the muscles and the joints. In this practice, the tapes are placed on the functional anatomical parts of the body—on the hurting muscle or joint area. Tape also is used in the treatment and prevention of sports injuries and helps stimulate the free flow of lymph fluid.

What does "kinesio-taping" mean?

The word *kinesio* comes from the Greek word *kinesis,* which means movement. The word *tape,* in medical usage, means sticky bandage. Kinesio-taping therefore means a therapeutic treatment method that uses sticky bandages to support movement. The bandages need to be flexible to allow for joint and muscle movement because their therapeutic effectiveness is dependent on the stimulation provided by movement, which helps to ease or eliminate the pain.

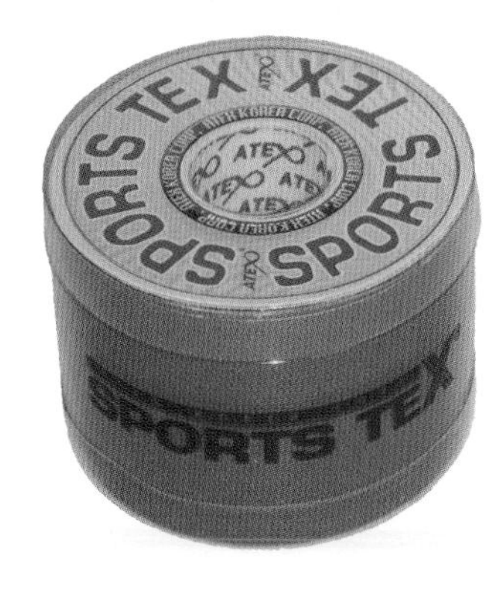

The tapes can be purchased in pink, blue, or tan cotton. The tan tape is energetically neutral, while the pink is associated with warmth and the blue with coolness.

What Is the Basis of Acutaping?

Acutaping is based on the knowledge and perceptions found in traditional Chinese medicine, acupuncture, and osteopathy.

The knowledge, perceptions, and therapeutic methods that come from the study of traditional Chinese medicine, acupuncture, and osteopathy are significantly different from what is found in Western medicine, and their use requires a thorough and additional training that rests in the hands of specialized doctors and therapists.

In conjunction with the use of flexible tape bandages applied in kinesio-taping, it is also possible to use this traditional knowledge in acutaping, a new treatment method that has a lot of advantages.

We do not regard acutaping to be in competition with acupuncture, acupressure, Chinese medicine, or osteopathy, but as an additional sensible treatment method that can enhance, in many cases, the effectiveness of other therapeutic methods. Moreover, the patient is able to become actively involved in the therapy because acutaping makes self-treatment possible. Most significantly, this especially encourages a positive partnership-oriented attitude to treatment that is, in our opinion, just as important for the healing process as the treatment itself.

Important!

The basis and application of acutaping

Acutaping therapy involves knowledge of acupuncture and Chinese medicine. This means that the therapist who decides where to best place the acutape for any given ailment must have a thorough training—in at least acupuncture, even better in traditional Chinese medicine—and a working knowledge of functional anatomy and osteopathy.

Once specific placement directions have been provided, though, the tape used in acutaping—which is affixed in a manner similar to kinesio-tape—is easy for the layperson to handle.

The Influence of Chinese Medicine

Chinese medicine is a holistic healing method that has been used for 3,000 years. Its origins can be seen in the talks that China's Yellow Emperor had with his personal physicians. In these discussions, the foundation for the development of a logical concept having to do with the prevention and treatment of illnesses was established and the illnesses got distinctive names that describe every ailment very precisely. A headache is characterized, for example, by a name that depends on the specific kind of headache and the nature of its occurrence, such as "piercing headache in the front part of the head" or "dull headache in the back of the head." These distinctive names also lead people to understand that different headaches might have different causes.

In its beginnings, Chinese medicine was clearly a departure from the practices of ancient shamans, who believed that illnesses were caused by bad spirits and that people had to go after these spirits to retrieve their good health.

Yin and Yang

The essential philosophical basis of Chinese medicine is found in the concept of yin and yang. The monad (Latin *monas,* from the Greek *monás,* meaning "simple" or "unit") symbolizes the indivisible union of two pairs of contradictory opposites, yin and yang. The yin and yang concept is based on the dualistic principle of order that brings together contradictory principles and conditions. So yin and yang can stand for night and day, moon and sun, earth and sky, dark and light, cold and warm, matter and energy, or stillness and activity. The essence of this principle of order is a totally value-free vision of the contradictory conditions. Therefore, in Chinese medicine yin and yang are never described moralistically as good or bad but are considered to be equally valued aspects of one unity. This can be explained with the example of day and night. We associate sun, warmth, and activity with the day and darkness, cold, and stillness with the night. If night did not exist and the sun was shining for twenty-four hours a day, the term "day" would have a totally different meaning. Because our perception of day is totally connected with the existence of night, it is also connected with the existence of a growing darkness. On the one hand, night and day are so very different they eliminate one another; on the other hand, they cannot be comprehended without each other. Another contradictory pair is joy and sorrow. To feel joy and to have the experience of a heartfelt happiness is only possible because we have the experience of sorrow. Whoever has never had an experience of sorrow feels that joy is boring.

The concept of yin and yang is essential in traditional Chinese medicine and its perception of illness and health. In Chinese medicine, being healthy means that yin and yang are in equilibrium. Illness results when the balance falls more to the side of either yin or of yang. When it moves more to the yang side, it is called yang plenty; when it moves to the yin side, it is called yin plenty. Next to plenty, there is also emptiness. With an empty condition, a patient has lost a lot of energy, so he or she is exhausted

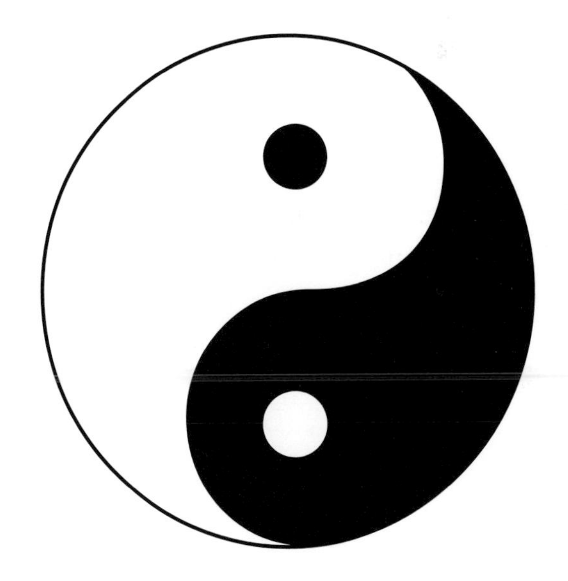

Yin and yang symbolize the harmony of the opposites.

because of a chronic disease, tired, and without a drive to do things. The framework of such a condition of emptiness can be a matter of a relative plus of yang or of a relative plus of yin.

The Five Elements

In contrast with practitioners of modern Western medicine, who understand and treat the human body exclusively in terms of its anatomy and physiology, ancient Chinese Taoist monks developed a medical system that links the human body to the cycles of nature that surround it. Traditional Chinese medical practitioners follow these Taoist principles to this day when diagnosing and treating people with health problems.

The Chinese laws of creation and control establish relationships among five phases of *chi,* or energy. These energies are represented in multiple interlocking cycles including: 1) five seasons of the year—spring, summer, Indian summer, fall, and winter; 2) five phases of creation—becoming, growing, ripening, harvesting, and perishing (or becoming dormant); 3) five natural elements—wood, fire, earth, metal, and water; and 4) five pairs of internal organs in the body—liver/gallbladder, heart/small intestine, spleen/stomach, lungs/large intestine, and kidneys/bladder. Thus the liver, for example, is linked to the element wood, the season spring, and the sprouting of new growth, while the heart is associated with the element fire, the season summer, and the time of blossoming.

Each element also has both positive and negative emotions associated with it. The positive emotion for the wood element is kindness but its negative emotion is anger. Thus an imbalance in the liver can manifest itself in a person's short-tempered, irascible mood. This way of perceiving the world may seem strange

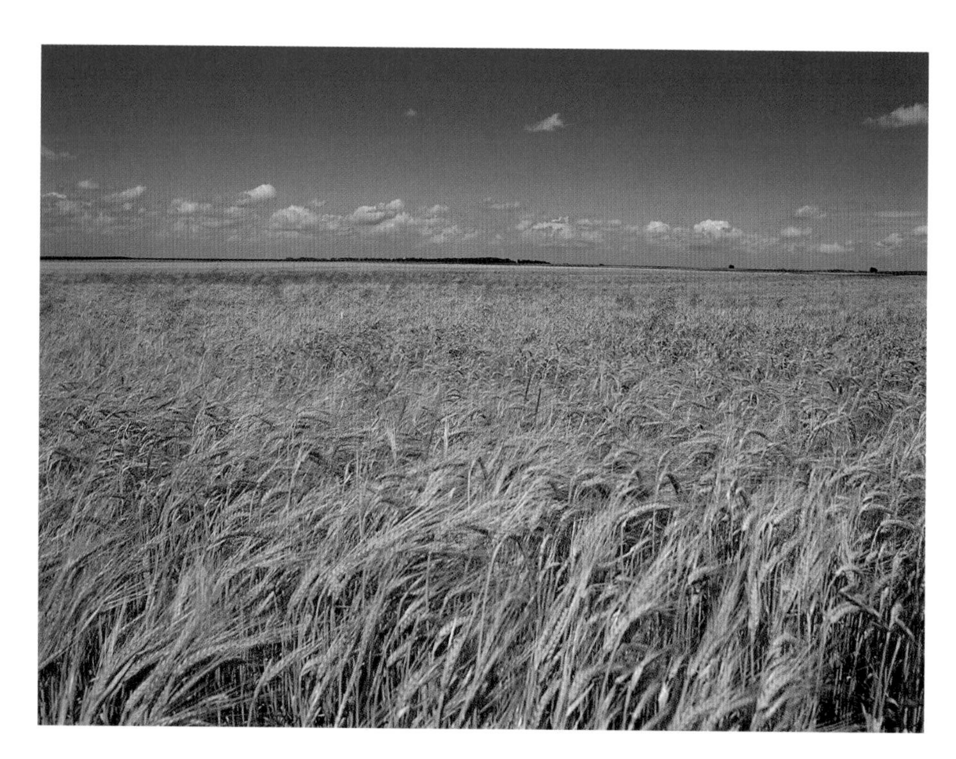

The circle of creation: becoming, growing, ripening, harvesting, and perishing

to our modern Western sensibilities, but our language shows that our ancestors were more in tune with this holistic view. The English word "liverish" means peevish, irascible, or short-tempered, and the archaic word "splenetic" means given to melancholy. In the Taoist system, the negative emotion associated with the spleen is depression.

In the Taoist cycles of creation and control, each season in the cycle is considered to be the "mother" of the season that follows it. So spring is the mother of summer and fall is the mother of winter, and so forth. The human organs associated with each season are considered to have similar relationships with one another. So the liver is considered to be the mother of the heart, the heart the mother of the spleen, and so forth. The traditional Chinese medical practitioner keeps these relationships in mind when treating energy imbalances in the organs. If an organ is too yin—too cold, weak, or deficient in energy—the practitioner will work to strengthen its mother organ on the premise that any mother with an excess of strength will naturally pass her excess energy on to her child. Conversely, if an organ is to yang—too hot, congested, or full of energy—the practitioner will take some energy from its child organ to stimulate the natural flow of energy from mother to child, thus balancing out the excess yang energy of the mother organ.

Practitioners of traditional Chinese medicine have several methods for diagnosing energy blockages and imbalances within the body. One diagnostic method is reading the pulses in the wrists. Each organ has a specific pulse associated with it. Indeed Taoists consider the pulses to be the sound of blood leaving the organs. By feeling for the pulse at specific points on the right and left wrist, the practitioner can ascertain the relative health of each organ system. Another method of diagnosis is to study the appearance of the tongue. Various areas of the tongue are linked to specific internal organs. For example, the left side of the tongue reveals the state of the liver, the right side the state of the gallbladder, and the tip of the tongue the state of the heart. The color, moisture, texture,

TAOIST RELATIONSHIPS BETWEEN HUMANS AND NATURAL CYCLES

Quality	Element				
Wood	Fire	Earth	Metal	Water	
Phases of creation (or sprouting)	Becoming	Blossoming	Ripening	Harvesting (or becoming dormant)	Perishing
Seasons	Spring	Summer	Indian Summer	Fall	Winter
Human organs Gallbladder	Liver/ intestine	Heart/Small Pancreas)/ Stomach	Spleen (and intestine	Lungs/Large Bladder	Kidneys/
Emotions	Kindness/Anger	Love/Hate Anxiety	Openness/ Depression	Courage/ Fear	Gentleness/

and coating on each part of the tongue gives the experienced practitioner valuable information about the relative health of the associated organ. Taking the pulses and studying the tongue are only two methods of diagnosis. The experienced practitioner of traditional Chinese medicine has a number of other diagnostic tools in his or her repertoire.

The Influence of Acupuncture

In the Taoist view of the human body, the life energy, or chi, runs throughout the body primarily within fourteen energy pathways called channels or meridians. Seven of the meridians are considered to be yin channels and seven of them are yang. Twelve of the meridians work together in pairs and are directly related to the internal organs. These six pairs of organ meridians were originally known as the "six great Heaven and Earth channels." The paired yang meridians are Bladder/Small Intestine, Gallbladder/Triple Heater (pelvis, abdomen, and chest), and Stomach/Large Intestine. The paired yin meridians are Kidney/Heart, Spleen/Lung, and Liver/Pericardium (also known as the Heart Constrictor). The two remaining channels, the Conception Vessel (yin) and the

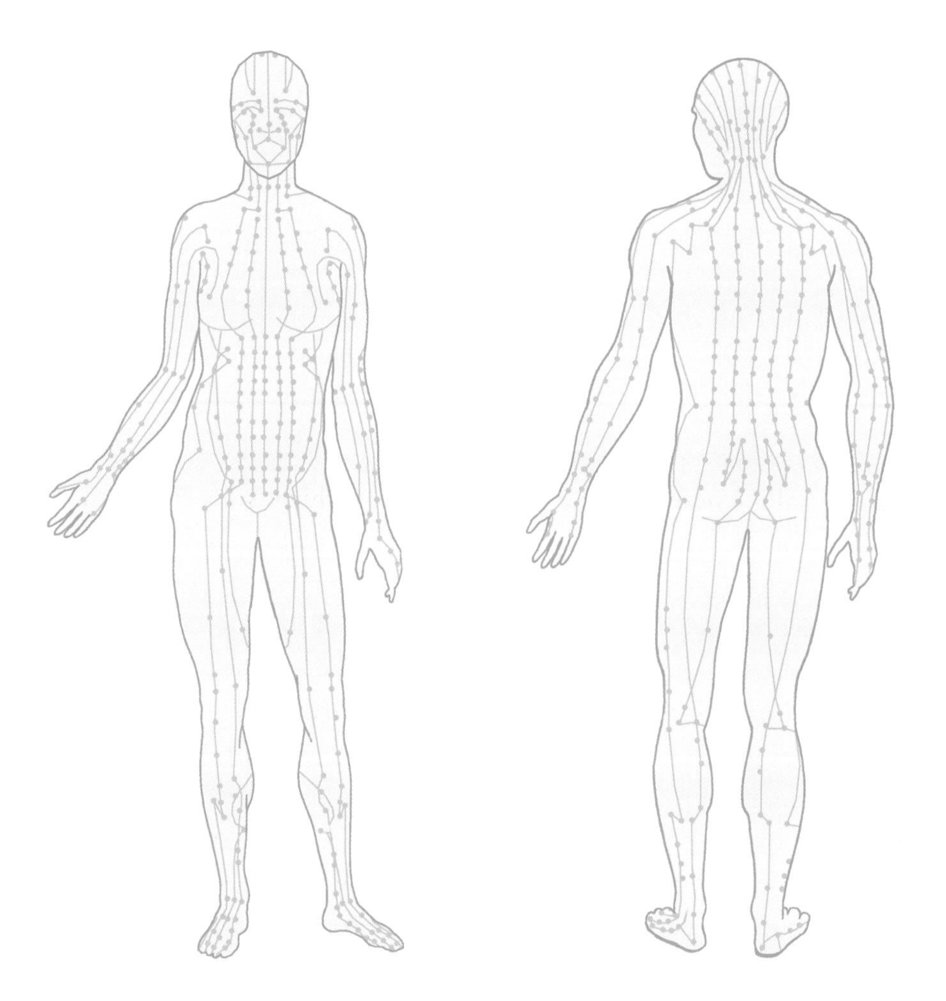

Location of meridian pathways and acupuncture/acupressure points in the body

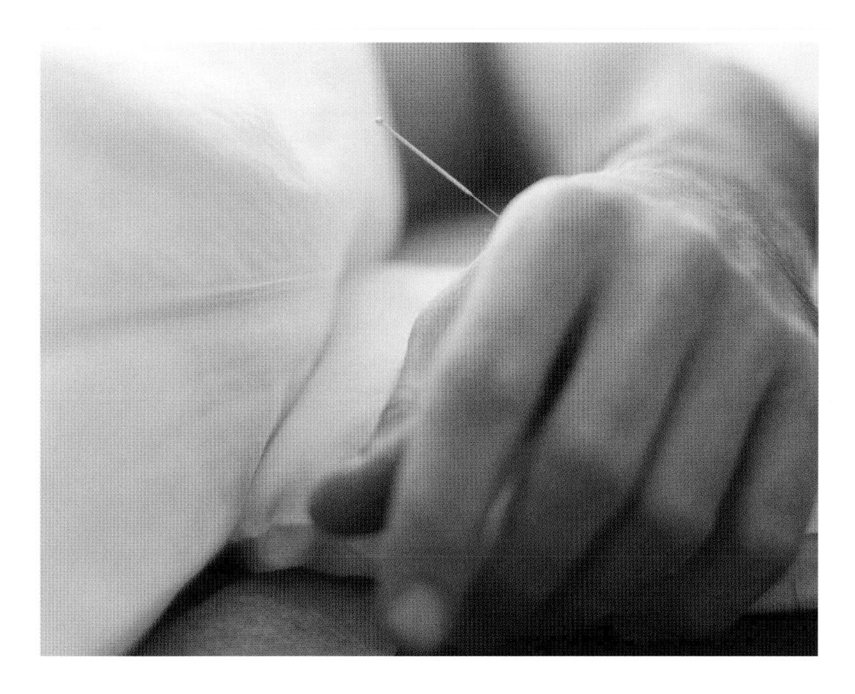

Acupuncture: A knowledge of traditional Chinese medicine provides a good foundation for acutaping.

Governing Vessel (yang) run up the front and back of the body at the midline.

Along these energy pathways are numerous points where the energy comes closer to the surface of the skin. These points are known as acupuncture points. They can be stimulated with acupuncture needles or by using finger pressure (acupressure) to clear energy blockages from the meridians and ensure a free flow of balanced energy to all of the internal organs.

After a practitioner of traditional Chinese medicine has made a diagnosis, he or she can treat the ailment with acupuncture needles or acupressure massage, Chinese herbs, and recommendations for diet and exercise therapy. A practitioner who uses acutaping brings his or her entire knowledge of Chinese medicine and acupuncture to bear when deciding where to place the acutapes. In contrast to kinesiotaping, which simply places the tape over the painful muscle or joint, acutaping seeks to stimulate acupuncture points along the meridians to circulate healing energy within the body. All of the tape placements offered in the second part of this book have been developed with an eye to the principles of traditional Chinese medicine and acupuncture/acupressure.

The Influence of Manual Medicine and Osteopathy

"Manual medicine," which is the treatment of functional disorders using the hands, has a long tradition. Based on that approach, Andrew Taylor Still, M.D., developed osteopathy in the United States at the end of the nineteenth century. The word *osteopathy* means literally "any disease of bone," and Dr. Still used this word as the name of his system of therapy, also. In osteopathy, the different functional systems of the body are examined thoroughly, and any deviation from normal movement is described. Through manual adjustments made to the spine and joints, the body is encouraged to reduce the dysfunctional pattern.

As in Chinese medicine, osteopathy is based on a holistic understanding of the human being. In contrast with the schools of chiropractic that were developed from the teaching methods of the Palmer brothers (the founders of chiropractic who attributed dysfunctions primarily to trauma, toxins, and thoughts), osteopathy involves a philosophy based on five biological principles that affect one another. When they are in harmony with one another, a person has achieved the condition that we call physical and psychological health.

The Five Principles of Osteopathy

1. Structure and function
2. The power of self-healing
3. The body as an entity
4. The circulation of the blood
5. The patient, not the illness

1. **Structure and function:** Structure and function act reciprocally with each other. If body structures such as joints, muscle groups, and organs are injured, it affects their ability to function. Such injuries also can lead to the disturbance of other body structures as well as broader sorts of dysfunction. An injury to a joint, for example, can affect not only its functional ability to move but can also cause muscle strain to intensify in the whole joint in an attempt to protect the affected area, so that a bone actually can be displaced. Basically, this is an innate survival mechanism of the body that may be understood

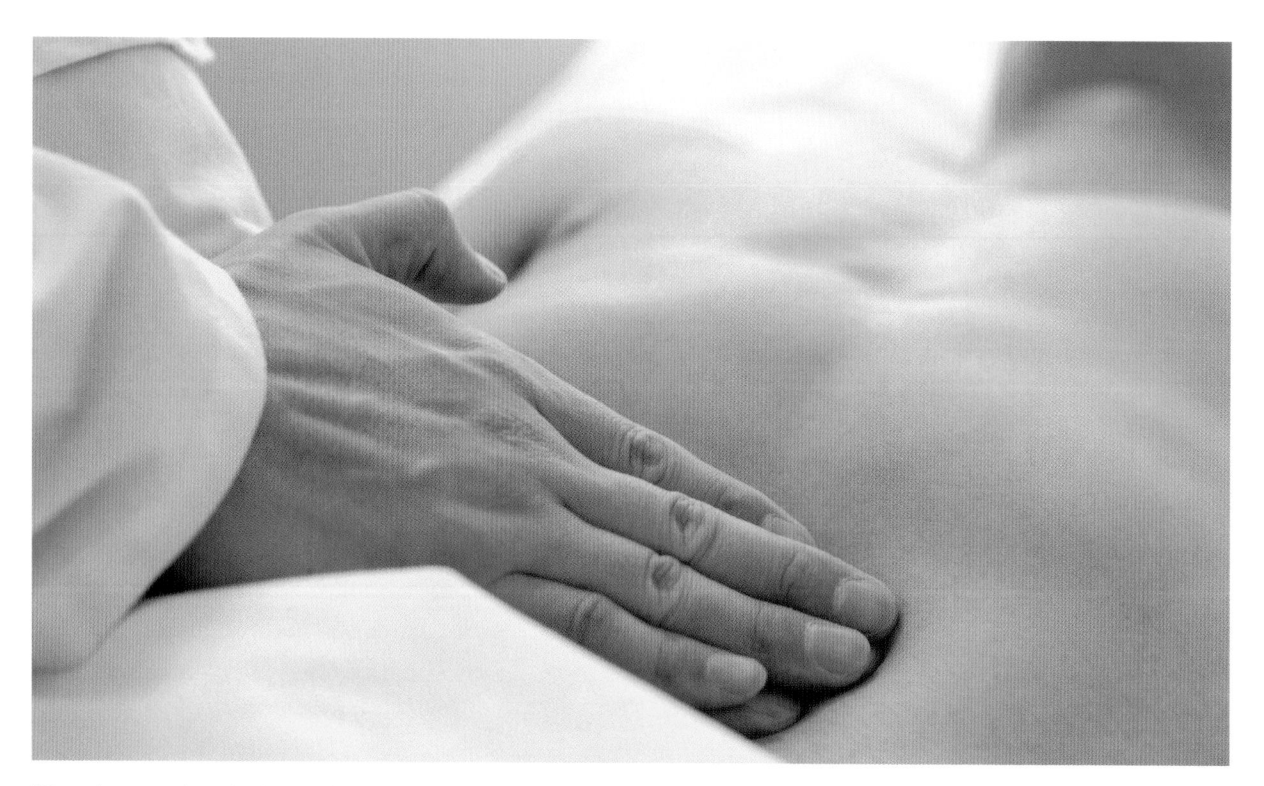

Disorders are treated with the hands.

in a positive light because it is an attempt to help the body compensate for an injury. However, if this attempt to compensate is not successful, it becomes—medically speaking—a *dis*compensation and starts making things worse. This means that, for all intents and purposes, a further problem begins to appear such as increased muscle tension, more pain, and greater restriction of movement. Because all parts of the body are in constant interaction through the connective tissue, bloodstream, and nervous system, a disorder in one specific part of the body can very quickly become a regional disorder; and its effects can be felt in the region of the inner organs as well.

2. **The power of self-healing:** This principle is based on the fact that when we are faced with illness, our bodies can generate the power to heal themselves. This process involves a permanent change within the organism. It is called adaptation. Particularly with functional, treatable disturbances, the body creates a compensation that neutralizes the effects of the disturbance and so protects the whole body against damage.

3. **The body as an entity:** Everything that has been said so far illustrates that the body is an entity. This entity is organized by the connective tissue that ensures the exchange of information throughout the body. For example, the connective tissue provides for the exchange of fluids that distribute hormones throughout the body, and it also carries information coming from the nervous system and immune system. The network of nerve fibers enables information to be sent back and forth instantly throughout the body. The sympathetic nervous system protects the body from lethal dangers, while the parasympathetic nervous system sends out signals that help the body to recover from injury or illness.

   The entity of the body uses a process of communication that is targeted dynamically and functionally. Every component of the body, including the bones, organs, bloodstream, nerve fibers, and others, fulfills a function that serves the body as a whole. At the same time, each and every component of the body depends on the functioning of the whole body. In other words, every part functions for the whole entity and through the whole entity in a harmonious togetherness in perpetual opposition to the outer world.

4. **The circulation of the blood:** The fourth and most important principle is the one having to do with the circulation of the blood. Blood transports all the secretions of the body and the chemical substances of nerve transmission as well. So the circulation of blood even influences our thinking. According to the philosophy of osteopathy, blood and fascia (connective tissue) are in direct exchange under the control of the nervous system. Thus, good blood circulation helps tissue nourishment, allows for the excretion of waste products, and prevents the blockage of the organs.

5. **The patient, not the illness:** This principle says that it is the patient who has to be seen and not the illness. The osteopath looks at the body as a whole entity of individual functions and functional processes in order to "feel" for blockages that affect these processes. His or her treatment then targets these blockages, loosens them up, and regulates the body flow in order to eliminate the disturbance and promote the natural healing process of the body.

Important!

Acutaping versus kinesio-taping

The difference between acutaping and kinesio-taping can be formulated in this manner: In acutaping, the knowledge and the rules of Chinese medicine and acupuncture/acupressure are used to translate Western symptoms and ailments into a Chinese clinical paradigm, and this perspective is used in the treatment, while kinesio-taping simply treats the area of pain directly. This is why acutaping is used for a broader scope of ailments than those treated with kinesio-taping.

How Does Acutaping Work?

It is not yet known precisely how the method works. All we can say is that we have been quite successful using this treatment, but we cannot explain exactly why.

In kinesio-taping and in acutaping, the tape bandages normally are applied to an area of the body that is stretched so that the muscles are taut. Because of its flexibility, the tape then adheres tightly to the skin during every movement of this area, which makes the surface skin that sticks on the tape lift away with the tape and move against the lower skin. It can be assumed that there is an effect similar to lymphoid drainage or a connective tissue massage. This certainly explains at least a part of the therapy's effectiveness.

In acutaping, the knowledge and experiences of practitioners of Chinese medicine, manual healing, and osteopathy are brought together in the therapeutic methods of taping. The acutape is applied to the muscle groups and acupuncture meridians that are associated with various illnesses. Their presence causes an irritation of the physical structures that lie beneath the tape—the skin, the loose connective tissue, and the tighter connective tissue (known in anatomical terms as superficial body fascia). As a result of the stimulating effects of this irritation, a normalization of the metabolism occurs. The normalization then starts the self-healing process of the body. Thus, through the way that it is used, both diagnostically and therapeutically, acutaping is very different from kinesio-taping, which has only a limited muscular and skeletal approach.

But the same rule applies for acutaping that applies for acupuncture and acupressure: Acutaping can only heal what is disturbed, not what is destroyed.

Examples of Acutaping Therapy

The following are three conditions that can be successfully treated using acutaping.

Headaches

The cause of a headache is usually a disorder of the muscles, ligaments, and joints in the neck and shoulder area. The precise cause can be pinpointed by a therapist. With kinesio-taping, the tape is placed along the course of the disturbed structures. In acutaping, we go one step further. From an ailment located in a particular muscle groups and skeletal region, further disturbance patterns can be deduced using the diagnostic methods of Chinese medicine. In the case of a headache, a disorder of the liver might be the cause. For example, the Chinese call another sort of ailment a "slime that congests the head," and it actually is connected to an illness of the spleen. Other possible further disturbance patterns could involve

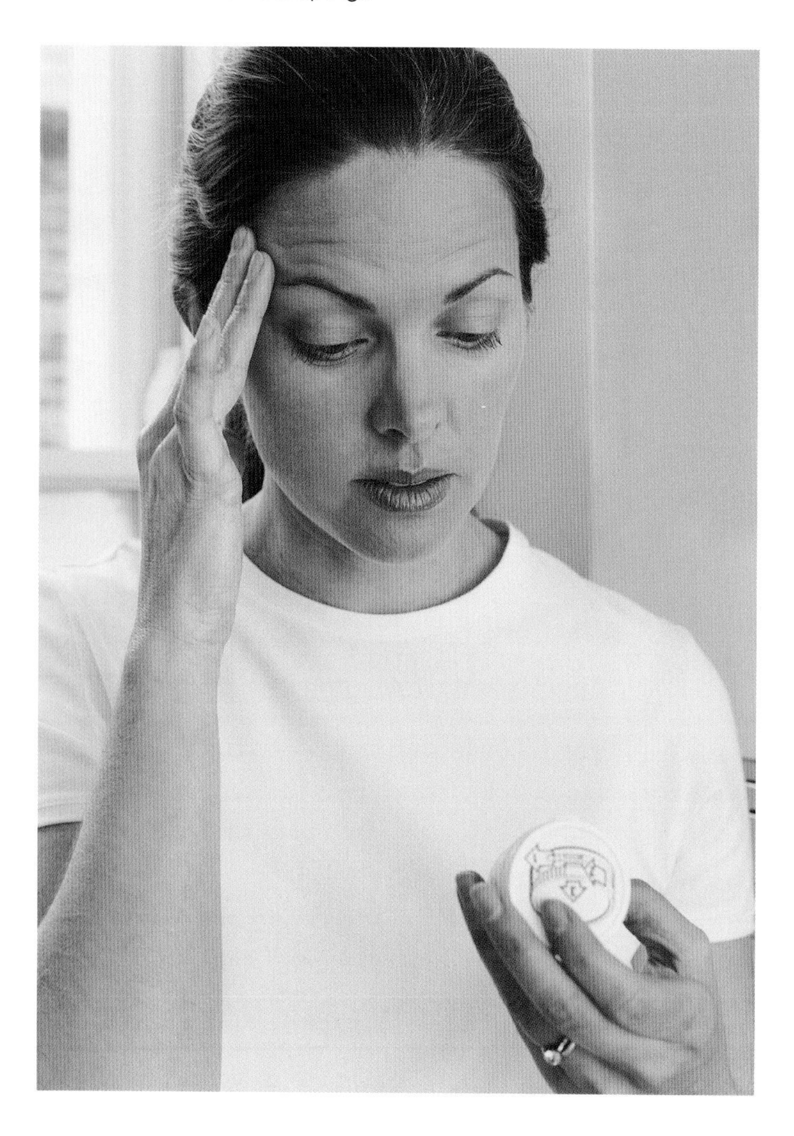

Acutaping helps with headaches.

a thinning of the blood or a disorder of the kidneys. This sort of additional knowledge can be taken into account when using acutaping, which means that special acupuncture points and acupuncture pathways are also taped.

Tennis Elbow

The principles of osteopathy also can be used in the treatment of tennis elbow. In contrast to kinesio-taping, in which the affected finger extensor muscle is treated, under the rules of osteopathy, the constant stretching of the irritated finger extensor muscle by the shortened finger flexor muscle is also treated.

Menstrual Pain

In kinesio-taping, the focus is on muscular and skeletal dysfunctions exclusively, so there is no therapy for menstrual ailments. On the other hand, the framework of acutaping is based on the diagnostic concepts of Chinese medicine and there is a well-developed therapy having to do with the treatment of menstrual ailments. The diagnosis of this condition involves a process of differentiating between "full" and "empty" conditions. In the full condition, there is too much energy in the body; in the empty condition, there is too little energy. With the help of this differentiation process, the disturbance patterns that cause the menstrual disorders be identified and treated. In addition, acutape can be affixed in such a way, following the rules of Chinese medicine, that a beneficial muscular and skeletal approach can also be taken into consideration.

Important!

Acutaping offers more

The previous examples showed that the approach to treating problems of the muscular and skeletal system in both methods—kinesio-taping and acutaping—is similar. In acutaping, however, the additional application of the rules of Chinese medicine, acupuncture/acupressure, and osteopathy offer a more complex, differentiated system of treatment possibilities. So the range of illnesses and injuries that can be treated using acutaping is much greater than with kinesio-taping.

Who Can Benefit from Acutaping?

Acutaping can benefit anyone who is suffering from chronic pain or wants to prevent it from happening. First, however, a doctor must be consulted to find the underlying cause of the pain.

Acutaping is a beneficial treatment for a variety of painful conditions such as joint and muscle pain or menstrual pain, and it is also effective in sports medicine.

To apply the techniques of Chinese medicine and acupuncture or acupressure along with acutaping, the help of a knowledgeable doctor or therapist is necessary. However, acutaping does offer the possibility of self-treatment, and in this book we will show you exactly how to do it. Patients with chronic knee pain can use acutaping regularly on their own or with the help of others. In many cases, the pain can be relieved and any inflammation can be reduced.

Acutaping also has been successful in the treatment of internal and gynecological problems, such as menstrual pain, and in the treatment of the various pains or discomforts that can occur during pregnancy.

Acutaping is now widely and successfully used for pain therapy in sports medicine. For example, prophylactic taping could be suggested for use during extremely strenuous activities such as marathons.

Various Indications for the Effective Use of Acutaping

With the help of acupuncture, we can positively influence the condition of certain body regions and functions. The same can also be said for acutaping. As with acupuncture and acupressure, acutaping can be used for many different applications, including the following:

- Abatement of acute and chronic pain
- Regulation of musculature (relaxing, restoring, invigorating)
- Regulation of organic disturbances from stress-related causes (relaxing, restoring)
- Regulation of immune reaction
- As an anti-inflammatory agent
- Improvement of blood circulation

Against What Sort of Pain Is Acutaping Effective?

Acutaping mainly is used in the treatment of acute and chronic pain conditions. (Again,

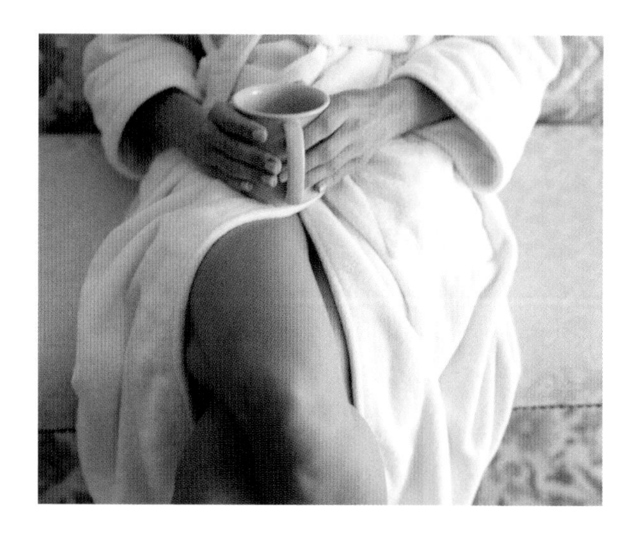

we want to remind you that it is of the utmost importance that you get a doctor's diagnosis before every treatment. If the examination shows that your disorder is in need of a broad range of treatment, acutaping can be included in this broader therapy.)

Disorders of the Structures of Movement

Acutaping has been used successfully in treating the following ailments:

- Joint pain
- Bruises of joints
- Strained muscles
- Sore muscles
- Headaches
- Shoulder pain
- Elbow pain
- Pain in the wrists
- Upper back pain (cervical spine)
- Middle back pain (thoracic spine)
- Lower back pain (lumbar spine)
- Pain of the coccyx
- Pain in the hips
- Pain in the knee
- Pain in the Achilles tendon
- Pain in the ankle joint
- Pain in the area of the calcaneus (heel bone)

Joint Pain

The tape is attached above the joint. For support, an additional strip of tape can be attached alongside the joint.

Bruises of Joints

Joint bruises are treated like joint pain.

Strained Muscles

The strained muscle first has to be stretched. If this is not possible due to pain, the tape has to be stretched out first and then taped on the muscle. The additional taping of the adjoining joint also has proved to be beneficial.

Sore Muscles

Acutaping has been beneficial in treating sore muscles. The tape is attached in the same manner as with a strained muscle.

Headaches

The treatment of headaches with different tapes can be very effective. Basically, headaches are designated as either tension headaches (located in the region of the neck and shoulder girdle) or vascular headaches (migraine or other cluster-attack conditions).

Most headaches are tension headaches. The tapes are applied according to the location of the pain. For headaches that go from the back of the head to the forehead or the eye, the cervical spine tape works well—maybe in combination with the cervical spine lymph tape, and the levator scapula muscle tape. If the headaches are felt in the temples, the cervical spine tape and the trapezius muscle tape, with its upper and middle part, is appropriate. If the headaches are more in the front part of the head, use the levator costarum (or scalenus) muscle tape, applied between the clavicle and the mastoid process, which is underneath the cranial bone and the earlobe.

Headaches that are caused by disturbances of the cervical spine also can be treated very successfully. Because these are often caused by

Does acutaping help with migraine headaches?

It is not possible to heal migraine headaches by using acutaping because they are caused by a pathological disorder (rather then a functional one) that will not be affected by using acutaping. It has been asserted that a migraine is an unusual neuromuscular illness that can be treated through intensive massage or kinesio-taping, but that seems highly dubious to us. On the other hand, any functional disturbances that might occur along with a migraine certainly can be successfully treated with acutaping.

functional disorders of the cranial joints and these problems can connect with functional disorders of the sacroiliac joint, the sacroiliac joint tape can be considered appropriate to use in treating these headaches.

Shoulder Pain

The pain is usually triggered when lifting the arm. To relieve the pain, the pectoral muscle in the chest (which is very often tense) and the biceps must be relaxed. In the framework of this pain treatment, we should generally use the trapezius muscle tape and the levator scapula muscle tape, the rotator cuff muscle tape, the pectoral muscle tape, the elbow joint extensor tape, the elbow joint flexor tape, the levator costarum (or scalenus) muscle tape, and the rhomboid muscle tape.

The various acutapes are not supposed to be applied simultaneously but one at a time in the location of the pain—where it hurts the most. In most cases, the trapezius muscle tape can be recommended as the starting point for the taping. One or two more tapes can be applied as well. If there is no reduction of pain, a trained therapist should be consulted. This is a general rule for all self-taping.

Elbow Pain

Elbow pain often is related to an irregular strain to the finger flexor and finger extensor muscles. This can lead to the well-known conditions known as "tennis elbow" or "golfer's elbow." Tennis elbow is characterized by pain at the point where the finger extensor muscle originates on the outer part of the upper arm bone. With golfer's elbow, the pain is on the inner side of the upper arm bone. These disorders often produce chronic irritations that also can become acute. Interestingly, the more acute the pain, the more effective the acutaping can be. With a chronic occurrence, there is very often a more complex disturbance pattern, mostly in the shoulder joint and the cervical spine area. This must be taken into account during treatment. The following tapes are applied in the treatment: finger and forearm extensor tape, finger and forearm flexor tape, elbow joint extensor tape, elbow joint flexor tape, and cervical spine tape.

Typically, pain associated with tennis elbow is caused by a pull in the finger and forearm flexor muscle. In such cases, it is recommended that the finger and forearm extensor tape and the finger and forearm flexor tape be applied simultaneously. If this does not work, then the elbow joint flexor tape and the cervical spine tape should be applied as well.

Pain in the wrists

The cause of this pain is often an irritation of the sinews in the area of the finger flexor and finger extensor muscles. The pain is also an expression of a general disequilibrium of this muscle area. So you treat the location where the pain occurs by applying the finger and forearm flexor tape and the finger and forearm extensor tape. In addition, you apply the cervical spine tape and, if there is a pain in the thumb, the thumb saddle joint tape. Many people who have this type of chronic pain either have or are developing arthritis. In the long term, treatment for arthritis is only likely to succeed if applied at the beginning of the illness.

Upper Back Pain (Cervical Spine)

Upper back pain often occurs along with headaches because trigger points in the muscles build up points of irritation that can be painful enough to radiate pain into other parts of the body. It is understood from osteopathy that disorders of the cervical spine can also cause secondary disorders. Treatment of the problems in the cervical spine alone will influence these secondary disorders but will not influence a preexisting primary disorder—the original cause of the pain. Only a professional therapist can sort out whether your pain is caused by a primary or a secondary disorder. However, you can successfully ease tension in the area around the neck and shoulder girdle yourself. This tension is often caused by awkward posture while working on the computer, and it can be treated very successfully by using acutaping. If this pain comes from twisting or stretching of the cervical spine, the cervical spine tape can be used, but if the pain is more to the side of the spine, it is recommended that you combine this with the levator scapula muscle tape also. Pain that occurs while turning the head can be treated with a combination of the levator scapula muscle tape, the levator costarum (or scalenus) muscle tape, and the trapezius muscle tape.

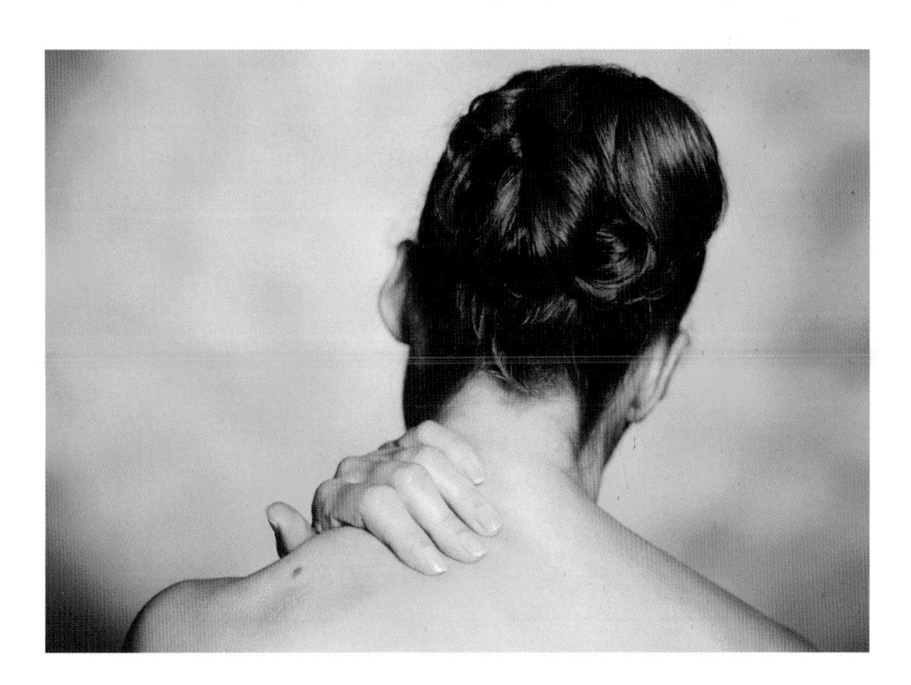

With acutaping you can easily relieve your own stress-related muscle tension.

Middle Back Pain (Thoracic Spine)

The thoracic spine consists of twelve vertebrae. Most human beings have functional disorders in various sections of the spine, but in many cases such disorders do not cause pain because the body can compensate well for them. However, if the bodily compensation becomes inadequate, the result is a discompensation, and this is associated with pain. In the area of the thoracic spine, there are a number of joints that can have functional disorders such as the joints between the thoracic vertebrae and the ribs and the two-finger-wide distance that lies beneath the spinous process of each vertebra. For instance, functional disorders of the rib joints have an influence on aspects of the nervous system. Dysfunction of the thoracic spine very often has the effect of negatively influencing the feedback to the organs of information that is essential for the sympathetic nervous system. Disturbances in the area of the thoracic spine are an expression of a major disorder that can be treated successfully as long as it is a functional and not a structural disorder. We know from Chinese medicine and especially acupuncture that there are important steering points along the acupuncture pathways in the area of the thoracic spine that can be influenced positively to work against a condition of illness. Acutaping of the thoracic spine region therefore can prevent a new occurrence of the pain—or at least delay it for a while. To treat the thoracic spine, you generally apply the thoracic spine tape and possibly also the rhomboid muscle tape, the pelvic bone muscle tape, or the hip and loin flexor tape.

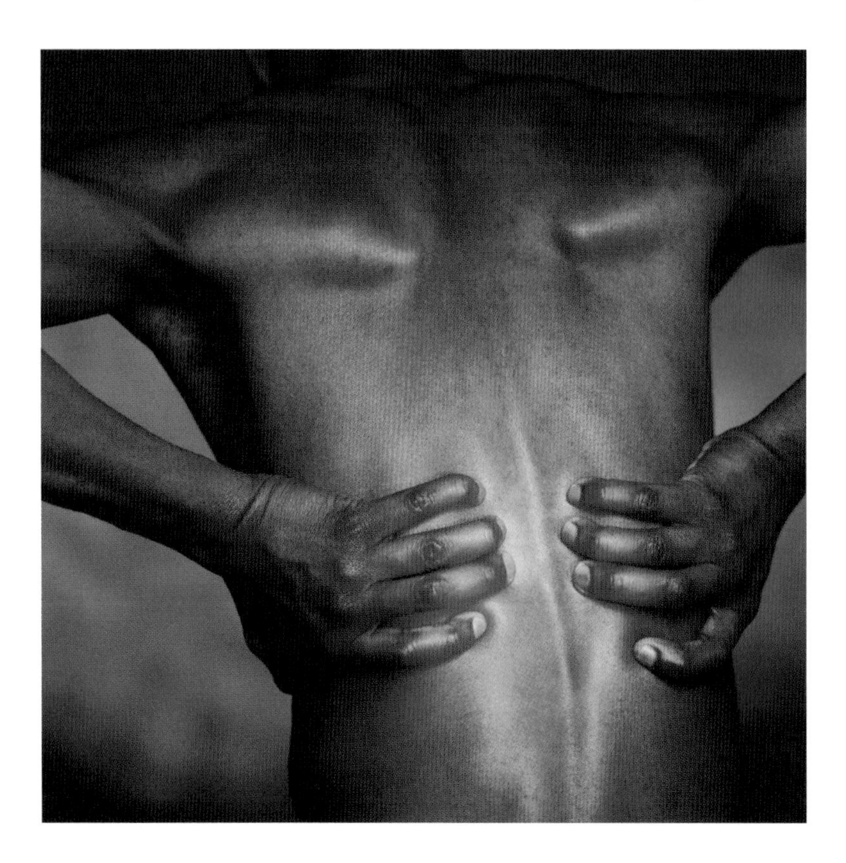

Acutaping helps relieve pain from a herniated disc.

Acutaping is effective in helping to prevent pain from everyday activities such as gardening.

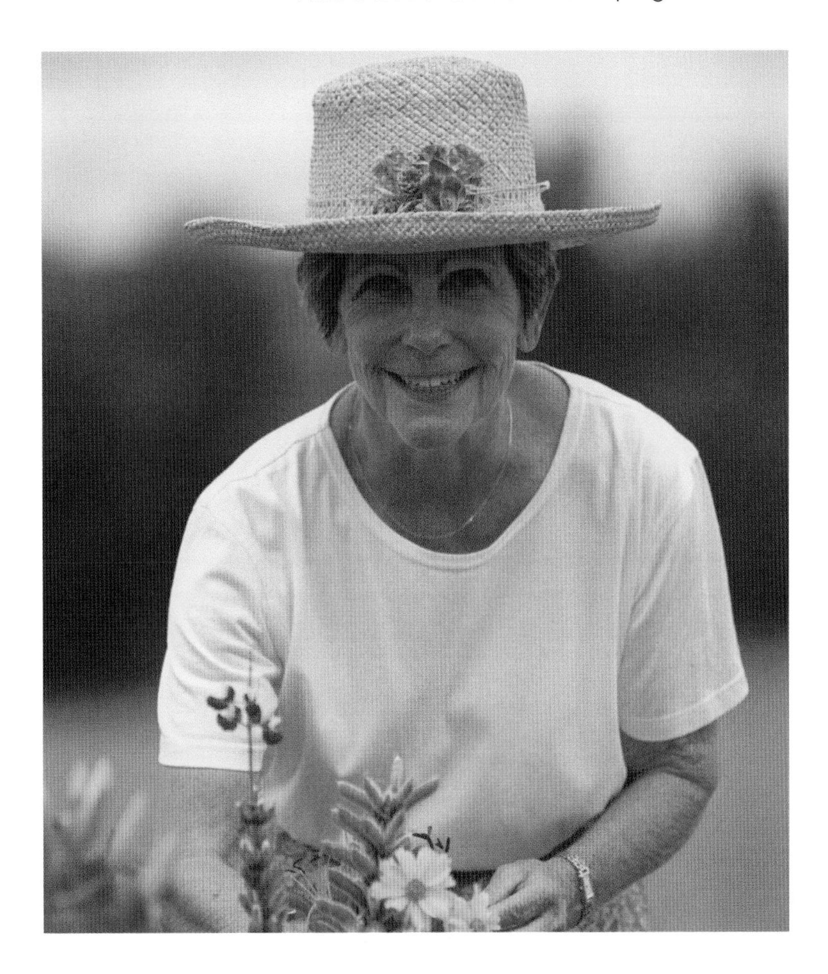

Lower Back Pain (Lumbar Spine)

Pain in this area is generally chronic pain. It usually reoccurs when the back is asked to bear an extra burden, such as an extended session of work in the garden. The pain is caused by a movement that compresses the spine, whether it's a sudden twisting motion or a sideways angled slant of the body. We speak of a group lesion if more than one of the vertebrae are affected. Very often, such compression in the lumbar spine can also cause a further disorder of the internal organs and lead to a more complex disorder. It is ideal to use acutaping as a follow-up to other treatment as well as using it as a preventive measure. Our recommendation would be to use the lumbar spine tape, the sacroiliac joint tape, and the pelvic bone muscle tape. If the pain radiates to the outer side of the hip joint, the lumbar spine star tape can be recommended. If the hip flexor muscle (the iliopsoas) that comes from the lumbar vertebrae to the hip joint is affected, the hip and loin flexor muscle tape should be used—especially if the pain radiates from the groin.

Pain of the Coccyx

For this, the lumbar spine tape, sacroiliac joint tape, and pelvic bone muscle tape are recommended, as they are with pain that occurs in the lumbar spine region of the back. For support,

Important!

Acutaping can be part of preventive and follow-up treatment of the spine.

Especially with backache, acutaping can be very successful as a both a preventive and a follow-up treatment. Disorders in the areas of the thoracic spine and lumbar spine are often caused by an overbearing stress from sports activity, working at the computer, or working in the garden. Acutaping can help to relieve these stresses. It also helps to prevent injury and works against certain disturbance patterns and ailments. In Part 2 of this book, acutaping is shown to help with follow-up treatment for spinal conditions, including postoperative support after surgery on a spinal disc.

stretched tape can be put on the coccyx area and in the top of the posterior fold between the buttocks.

Pain in the Hips

This pain can occur *symptomatically.* This means that the cause is not actually in the area of the hip itself but that the pain is instead a symptom of some other condition. Very often the pain comes from the lower back into the groin and the outer hip. Sometimes, pain caused by a disorder in the knee joint can be felt in the hip first. A visit to a professional therapist would be advisable for diagnosis of the source of the pain. If pain originates from the lumbar region, the following tapes can be used: lumbar spine tape, pelvic bone muscle tape, sacroiliac joint tape, and hip and loin flexor muscle tape. If the pain originates from the edge of the upper pelvic bone, use a combination tape (also called *pes anserinus* tape) for the sartorius muscle in the thigh, the hip joint abductor, and the inner part of the knee joint flexor. If the disorder originates in the posterior of the thigh and the pain radiates from there to the hollow of the knee, it is usually the result of too much stress on the muscle or of a muscle pull in the area of the reverse thigh muscle. In that case, the knee flexor tape can be used.

Pain in the Knee

Here you have to differentiate between functional disorders that occur around the kneecap and those that occur in the inner or outer side part of the knee. Disorders in the hollow of the knee are often caused by a pull in the reverse thigh flexor muscle. Irritation on the inner side of the knee joint often follows surgery on the meniscus or the ligaments or an operation on the knee itself. To avoid athletic injuries, the knee joint usually has to be taped with an eye to prevention. The acutape that is used to treat pain in both the inner and outer sides of the knee is the combination tape, which also is known as the pes anserinus (knee joint) tape. It provides treatment for pain in the sartorius muscle in the thigh, the knee flexor muscle on the inner side of the knee, and the hip joint abductor muscle. The use of this acutape to treat bruises on the inner and outer sides of the knee joint results in an anti-inflammatory effect and a lessening of pain.

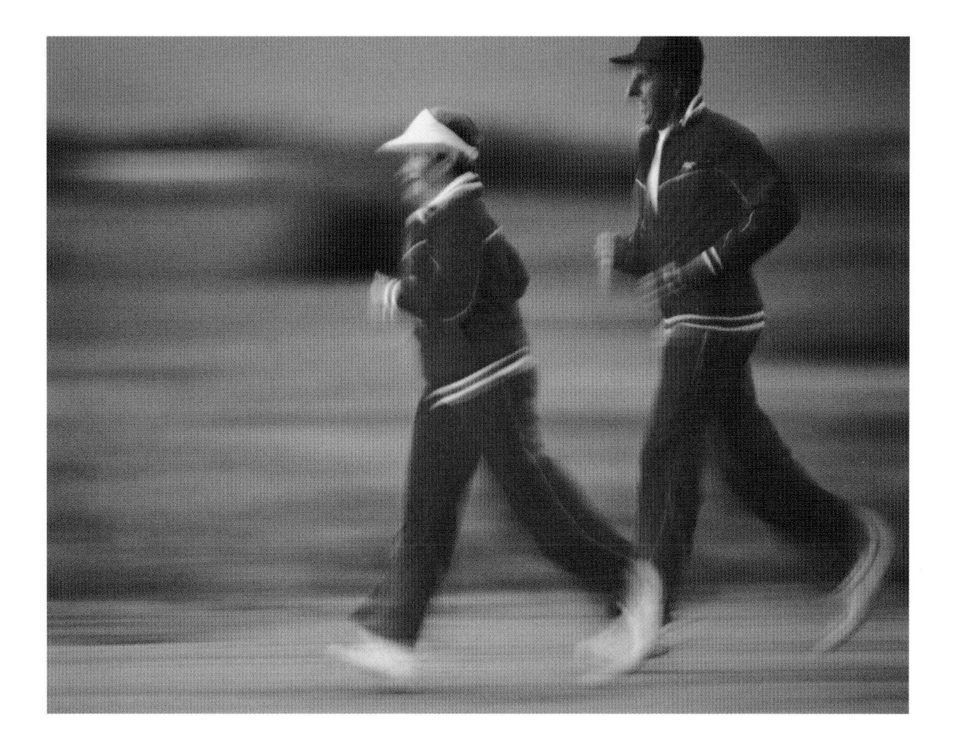

Runners often have problems with their Achilles tendons.

Pain in the Achilles Tendon and Ankle Joint

People involved in sports often have pain in their Achilles tendons. The reason for this is usually a problem with the shape of the arches of their feet or bad running shoes that do not provide enough arch support. So first of all, it is important to have an orthopedic examination. Functional disorders that are detected in the tarsal area often can be treated quite effectively with manual therapy. Any pain that still remains is very often of muscular origin. In such a case, the Achilles tendon and ankle joint tape is used. With this tape, the acupuncture points in the area of the Achilles tendon are stimulated, which helps relax the calf muscles and takes the stress off the Achilles tendon. The taping of the ankle joint at the same time enhances the effect of the Achilles tendon tape. This also helps with a sprain from a twisted ankle.

Pain in the Area of the Calcaneus (Heel Bone)

Pain in the area of the heel bone often occurs in a person with very high arches. This is a pain that usually has its origin in the tarsal area. It is important here to have a therapist loosen and relieve any functional disturbance of the tarsal bones. As a follow-up treatment, you can use the Achilles tendon and ankle joint tape—with the Achilles tendon tape attached only up to the middle of the sole of the foot.

Internal Illnesses

Many people have reported success in using acutape to treat the following illnesses:

- Stomachache
- Indigestion
- Chronic constipation
- Diarrhea

These problems of the digestive tract can be treated with the abdominal muscle tape (both rectus and oblique) supported with the lumbar spine tape. If acutaping is not successful, the treatment can be combined with acupuncture.

Pain during Pregnancy

Acutaping can help a lot during pregnancy, which can create many problems in the region of the lumbar spine or the belly. It is crucial that during pregnancy, any attempt at self-treatment be discussed and coordinated with a gynecologist. Effective treatment is possible for the following ailments.

Pain in the area of the belly: Pain in the belly region can be treated with lumbar spine tape using abdominal muscle tape (both rectus and oblique) as support.

Backache: Backaches happen often during pregnancy. Lumbar spine tape can help a lot here. With a backache that falls in the thoracic spine region, thoracic spine tape is recommended. If the problem does not fully respond to this treatment, you can also use the sacroiliac joint tape, though it might be helpful to have a therapist apply the tape the first time and coach your taping partner in how to apply it.

Vomiting (nausea) during pregnancy: Acutaping can help control vomiting during pregnancy. There are important acupuncture points in the area of the finger that affect nausea, so the finger and forearm flexor acutape is used. If this alone does not help, acupuncture or acupressure can be combined with the acutaping.

Further Disorders

Bruising: An acutape can be attached over the bruise, according to the direction of the underlying muscle.

Clearing the residual effect of scars (interference suppression): The interference supression of scars can be attempted with the help of different therapeutic possibilities. The options of subdermal injection of local anesthetics or treatment with acupuncture should only be done by a therapist. For interference suppression self-

Cellulite

The successful treatment of connective tissue weaknesses, such as cellulite, using acutaping is relatively new. A long-term treatment approach is necessary. Before attempting any self-treatment an experienced therapist should be consulted, but the local application of the basic tapes can be done by a layperson. These tapes are stretched as far as possible when applied. Where it is possible, the area in question should be stretched also so that the stretched tape is applied to stretched skin.

treatment by a layperson using acutaping, the length of tape should be stretched over the scar as far as it can be stretched and changed every two days.

Ringing in the ears (tinnitus): Acutaping can help lessen the ringing caused by tinnitus when used in conjunction with other therapeutic measures provided by a professional. You should use the cervical spine tape, the cervical spine lymph tape, the levator scapula muscle tape, the trapezius muscle tape, and the sacroiliac joint tape.

Dizziness: Dizziness can be treated by using the cervical spine tape, cervical spine lymph tape, levator scapula tape, trapezius muscle tape, and sacroiliac joint tape.

Acutaping in Sports Medicine

In different sports, various joints or muscle areas come under great stress. Depending on where the stress occurs, acutaping can be used therapeutically and preventively.

Acutaping offers a variety of specific preventive approaches for sports medicine—and for sports activity in general. With the preventive acutaping of muscles and joints under stress, much of the risk of injury can be avoided.

The method of kinesio-taping developed by Dr. Kenzo Kaze was first presented to the general public during the 1988 Olympic Games in Seoul, Korea. Some of the athletes on the Korean Olympic team attracted attention because of their colorful kinesio-tapes.

The advantage of flexible tape bandages over inflexible conventional tape bandages, which are designed to restrict movement, is that the elastic material does not inhibit natural movement, yet helps to improve the metabolism in the area of treatment. This is why the tapes are successful *prophylactically*—they prevent damage from happening. Still, it is important to remain alert for any recurring disturbance in the muscle area of joints, which can signal the onset of a serious condition of the affected joint. It is always important to consult a sports doctor or an orthopedist for help in trying to prevent sports-related injuries.

A given sport will put stress on a particular area of the body. The effect of this stress can be eased by using acutaping and taking care to not overstress the area. For instance, with sports such as tennis, squash, badminton, and golf that use backstrokes of the arm, the elbow joint is under stress. Along with the finger and forearm flexor and extensor taping, people who participate in these sports should also use a stretching exercise for the finger flexor muscle to prevent stressing the finger extensor muscle because stress in these muscles can lead to elbow pain. To be able to make a strong fist, the finger flexor and finger extensor muscles have to work together. Yet the finger extensor is prone to stress reactions because the muscle of the finger flexor is a lot stronger.

The region of the shoulder joint is also often under great strain during sporting activity. For example, if the upper thoracic spine is overworked in the repetitious lifting of the arm for the serve in tennis, it leads to less flexibility in the shoulder joint. To prevent this problem, the thoracic spine tape can be applied as a prophylactic measure.

The upper part of the lower rotator cuff muscle that lies on the shoulder joint is also prone to getting pulled. The rotator cuff acutaping can be used as a prophylactic measure. The same taping can be used to prevent pain in the biceps, if they are prone to being pulled as well, and also can prevent the possibility of an accompanying disorder in the elbow joint.

If there is a tendency for tension to build up in the area of the thoracic spine and lumbar spine, acutapes can be applied there as a prophylactic measure. This is recommended for exercise regimens on a treadmill or elliptical trainer.

For sports like tennis or handball (and also for activities like gardening) that involve rotation in the area of the lumbar spine, the lumbar spine region can be acutaped as a prophylactic measure.

Knee tape (especially for ailments around the knee cap) has proven effective for runners. For this area, it is important to always remember to do a sufficient amount of stretching for the thigh muscles.

Soccer and handball players very often have injuries to the area of the inner side of the knee and to the area of the adductor muscles, which are used for bending the knee. Here the combination tape for the sartorius muscle, the hip joint abductor muscle, and the knee joint flexor on the inner side has been used successfully.

Recurring or chronic disorders in the area of the Achilles tendon can be treated with the Achilles tendon and ankle joint tape. Runners, especially, should make sure that the heels are very tightly enclosed and well-cushioned in the running shoes so that they can be safeguarded from any possible strain of the ligaments, muscles, and joints during running. Get good advice on which shoes to buy!

Basically, you should make sure you always warm up and stretch the muscles well before any sports activity. Then the acutapes can be of further help—an additional support for muscles and joints.

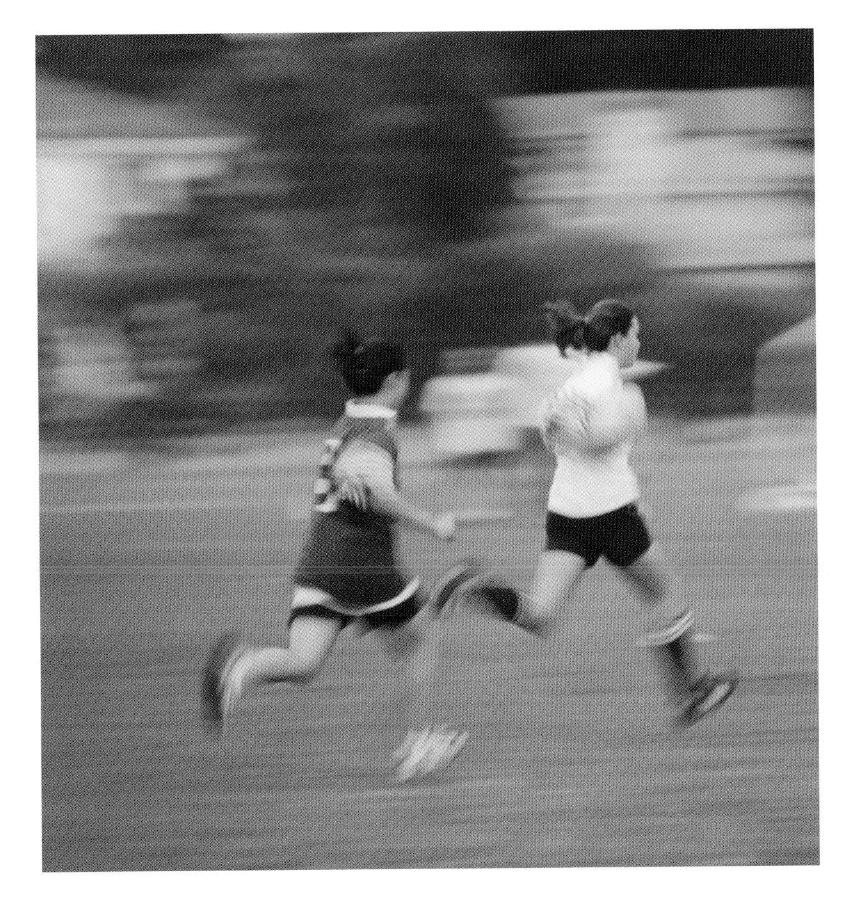

In sports medicine, acutaping has proven that it can be used effectively to prevent an ailment from developing.

When Not to Use Acutaping

A complex or a structural disorder can lead to conditions in which acutaping is of little or no help. For some illnesses, taping should not be used.

Acutaping is not a "cure-all." There are a number of reasons why taping may not be effective and conditions for which it should not be used at all.

If, after three or four sessions of acutaping, there is still no improvement in any ailment we have described, we urgently recommend that you consult your doctor or therapist. This is because there are a number of possibilities why taping might not be effective. If taping does not provide relief, further examination and diagnosis is necessary to determine the cause of your ailment. For example, it could be that the ailment is only one aspect of a more general illness you have. The primary cause could be a complex or a structural disorder that requires a more general approach to therapy. There are also other factors that could inhibit or prohibit the effect of the acutaping.

Complex or Structural Disorders

If there is a complex or even a structural disorder (such as a chronic illness), acutaping should not be the only therapy that is used. If, for example, a backache is caused by hip joint abrasion, taping alone can be of little help. However, it can be used in tandem with whatever medically appropriate therapy is decided upon for treatment, such as drugs for pain relief, movement therapy, physiotherapy, or relaxation therapy.

An Example: Elbow Pain

A pain in the elbow (such as tennis elbow) can be caused by momentary overload originating in the finger extensor muscle at the outer upper arm bone. However, an overload on the biceps or a pulled muscle also can cause a disturbance of the flexibility of the radial head joint at the outer part of the elbow, which can be the cause of the pain.

In addition, functional disturbances of the lower cervical spine radiate pain into the area of the elbow joint, and certain shoulder joint disturbances also cause pain in the elbow. That means that an acutape positioned at the disturbed elbow joint will not be effective when the origin of the disorder—the area of the cervical spine, the shoulder joint, the biceps, or the radial head joint—is not treated also. These causes of pain can only be diagnosed by a doctor or therapist.

Other Factors Pertaining to a Disorder

If there has been no progress in healing after using acutape, even though there has been a correct medical diagnosis, the factors of the disorder have to be understood in terms of naturopathy. Such a disorder could be caused by an inflamed tooth, a chronic inflammation of the sinuses, or even a psychological disturbance.

If a psychological factor is causing tension in the shoulder and neck area, acutaping can help lessen the tension, but due to the underlying psychological disturbance and the muscle stresses it provokes, the ailment can reoccur. As in all such cases we have mentioned, long-term therapeutic success is likely to happen only if the disorder that caused the ailment is treated. Such disorders and their causes are listed below.

Regulatory Blockages/Reactive Stiffness

The term *regulatory blockages/reactive stiffness* comes from naturopathy. It means the body cannot respond to subtle changes in stimuli because of a systemic condition that blocks its normal response. In this case, acupuncture and acutaping usually cannot help. Some other therapy must be used to remove the regulatory blockage.

Acidity

Naturopathic medical theory maintains that regulatory blockages can be caused by acidity in the body. It is very easy to determine acidity: Do a pH measurement of your urine and saliva for several weeks. You can get paper pH test strips and a pH index in any pharmacy. First, put the pH strip in your mouth and wet it with saliva. The paper strip will change color. Compare the color of the strip with the index, where you can find the number that corresponds to that color. Write down the number in a notebook. Then, put a new pH-paper slip in a sample of your urine and check the color of that paper strip with the index. Write down that number as well. Do this every morning and every evening for several weeks. You should also keep a record in your notebook of your eating habits—write down all the food and drink that you take in. Average urine and saliva numbers under a pH of 6.5 suggest excess acidity. An experienced doctor of naturopathy can help you establish the treatment protocols you need and start you on a course of therapy to reduce your acid levels.

Warning: Self-treatment of excess acidity must not be attempted. With some acid-related ailments that involve the formation of stones (such as kidney stones), you can actually worsen your condition.

Scar Formation

In naturopathy, scars are seen as capable of causing disturbances throughout the body. You can clear up the systemic effects of scars (which is called interference suppression) by using acutaping.

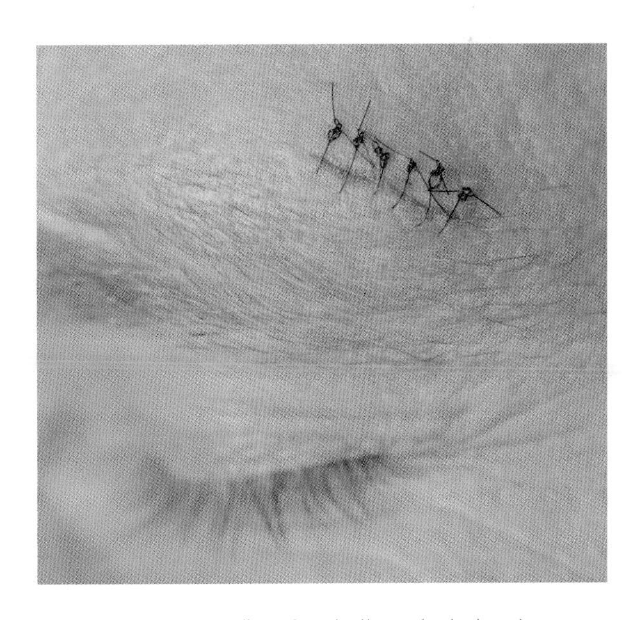

Scars can cause disorders in the whole body.

When Acutaping Is Not Advised

As stated before, acutaping is no panacea. For some ailments, taping does not help and for others it is even dangerous. Patients with certain illnesses simply should not be acutaped. Such illnesses are:

Clinical Patterns That Have Not Been Cleared by Medical Doctors

It is very important to have any ailment and its cause diagnosed by a medical doctor, before treatment with acutaping.

Blood-Clotting Disorders

Some patients take medicine to prevent the clotting caused by a circulatory disorder. In extreme cases, acutaping may cause hemorrhaging. Therefore, patients who are taking anti-clotting medicine must consult with their medical doctor before using any type of acutaping treatment.

Patients with a genetic disorder that prevents the clotting of blood, such as hemophilia, should not be acutaped.

Psychological Problems

Every illness has its psychosomatic expression. This means that a treatment of a psychological condition by using acutaping should be possible and desirable. However, as with many instances of energy medicine including acupuncture and acupressure massage, the treatment can at first cause a worsening of the situation. This has to be taken into consideration. With profound psychological illnesses, such as depression or psychosis, a medical specialist must be consulted before attempting therapy with acutaping. The temporary worsening could be dangerously destabilizing for an acutely ill patient. Such a patient would need the supervision of a medical professional for any course of treatment.

Acutape: Information and Tips

In this chapter, you'll find lots of information and tips about acutaping to help you make the right choices and to help you with the proper handling and practical use of the acutape.

What are the highest quality tapes made of, and what do they look like? Can you take a shower or a sauna with the acutape still on? How often do the tapes need to be changed? How long should a treatment with the tape last? How do you avoid mistakes that can lead to failure? The answers to these questions and more can be found here.

Description of the Acutape

- The acutape is made of flexible cotton fabric, with no latex. Lengthwise, it can be stretched to 130 percent or 140 percent of its normal size. Crosswise, the elasticity is about 10 percent.
- There is an acrylic glue on one side of the tape. Acrylic glue is thermoplastic, which means that it expands when heated and constricts when cooled.
- The glue has been put on the tape in waves so that air can permeate the adhesive area and the skin under the tape can breathe.
- During use, the tapes are also water permeable, which means that they can be left on when you are in the shower or the sauna. The tape will allow the water to pass through it.
- Because it is water permeable, the tape does not block any moisture released through the skin.
- Sweat underneath the tape is not a problem, but immersion in salt water is not good for the tapes and will make them fall off the skin fairly quickly.

Some Practical Tips

In the following section, you will find some information and tips that you should consider carefully when taping. They will insure the success of the acutaping treatment as well as its comfort and ease of handling.

The condition of the skin: The skin in the area where the tape is attached should be dry and not greasy. If necessary, wash the skin with a moist cloth and then dry it with a towel.

What to do about hairiness: Men who are quite hairy tend to have a problem with the stickiness of the tape. Clipping the hair a little shorter with a pair of scissors is a good idea, but shaving it is not recommended because it might cause skin irritation that can become inflamed underneath the tape.

Helping hands: When there are a number of muscles involved in the areas being taped or when the tape location is in a hard-to-reach area, you will find you are not able to apply the tape on your own and you will need the help of a partner.

Preliminary stretching: Before you start taping, you should stretch the areas of the body that are to be treated. This means that the point of muscle extension and the point of muscle origin have to be at the farthest possible distance from each other. For example, to apply the finger and forearm flexor tape properly, the wrist has to be brought into a hyperextended position so that the muscle at the elbow joint is stretched. With the elbow straight, the wrist must be bent up as far as possible and the forearm twisted toward the little finger.

Measurement and preparation of the tape: With the area to be treated properly stretched, the tape is laid out on that area so that it can be cut to the proper length. To avoid the tape unraveling at the edges it's best to round off the corners with scissors before attaching it. Then you peel a little of the paper backing from one end of the tape.

Attaching the tape: Don't forget to do a preliminary stretch of the muscles! To continue with the example of the finger and forearm flexor tape, the end of the tape is attached on the location of the finger flexor, in the area of the inner upper arm bone. The rest of the tape is taken off the backing paper without bending or stretching the tape, so that it runs along the muscle under the arm to the palm of the hand. Then the tape is attached to the skin, starting with the middle of the tape and going to the ends. Just as with putting on wallpaper, you need to be careful that the attachment is not too tight, so that the tape does not give easily or wrinkle. After half an hour, due to the warmth of the body, the glue takes full effect and the tape will stick more tightly.

Changing the tape: The tape can remain on the skin for three to seven days. Under normal circumstances the tapes will easily stay on that long and generally do not come off during showering.

Rare but possible side effects

In rare cases side effects can occur, mostly due to the irritation of the skin where the tape is attached. Side effects include:

Itching

Patients who have very sensitive skin can develop a redness of the skin or an itching. This is very rare, and the tapes can simply be removed.

Allergic Reaction

There are very seldom any allergic reactions. We treat a lot of people with neurodermatitis and other chronic skin diseases, and even in our practice, allergic reactions to the tape are very rare. If a mild allergic reaction such as redness or itching does occur, then the tape must be removed. Normally any mild allergic reaction wears off after two or three days. Only occasionally is medical treatment necessary. A very strong allergic reaction, such as hives or swelling, will not necessarily go away, however. If you have a stronger allergic reaction, you should always consult your doctor.

Early deterioration of the tape: Depending on the consistency of sweat, the tape *can* fall off earlier. However, you can put a new one on to replace it without any problems. Tapes on hands or feet do tend to come off earlier. Putting an extra tape across another can help. Also, it helps to wear thin socks over tape on the feet both day and night. During the night socks are helpful to keep the tape from coming off because of unconscious movements of the body while sleeping.

What to do if you experience pain when you remove the tape: If it hurts when you take off the tapes, you should moisten them first before removing them.

Acutape Colors

The tapes can be purchased in pink, blue, or tan cotton. The color of the acrylic glue is the same for all three tapes.

Some patients say that when they use the pink tape they experience a distinct feeling of warmth; other patients say that they feel coolness when they use the blue tape. We are acquainted with this sort of sensation from our experience with light therapy. Though this phenomenon when using acutape has not been proved, you can experiment with the different tapes to see if you experience varying sensations based on tape color.

Blue, Pink, and Tan Tape—Tips for Therapy

You have to test to find out how you react to each color of the tape. It may very well be that one color of tape is uncomfortable. If that is so, you have to remove it and use a different color tape. To start, you should use the following guidelines:

Blue Tape: For ailments in which the skin is bright red and/or feels hot, you should use the "cooler" blue tape. With acute conditions, such as swelling in the joints, the blue tapes are effective.

Pink Tape: Though heat feels comforting, chronic pain such as that found in persons with arthritis does not respond well to actual heat in the long run. Use the "warmer" pink acutape instead. According to the Chinese understanding, chronic pain accompanied by an ongoing, dull "pulling" sensation of discomfort indicates that there is a lack of energy. The pink acutape has been effective for these conditions, and some patients praised the warm feeling they felt with this color tape.

Tan Tape: The tan acutape can be used any time. From our experience, it can be considered energetically neutral.

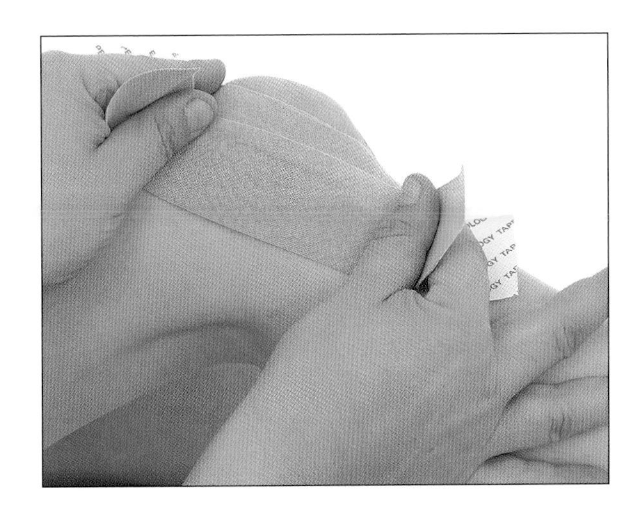

What Areas of the Body Can Be Treated?

This depends mainly on the primary source of the pain. Acutaping placements have been developed so that they cover or include the primary area of pain. The therapist who treats you will determine what other areas need treatment to ensure success. The rule is that although this book can give you valuable information and guidance for self-treatment, it cannot replace the essential value of a therapist's understanding and knowledge when diagnosing the source of your pain.

Duration of Therapy

For chronic disease, you should estimate that the duration of treatment will be up to several weeks long. Five- to ten-day treatment protocols, spaced a week apart, are sensible. For acute illness, three to five treatments should be enough. As a preventive measure, the tapes can be applied before sporting activities and removed afterward.

How to Prevent Failure

Failure when using acutaping can usually be prevented by having a doctor examine you first. If the examination shows that you have a basically remediable functional disorder, treatment that includes acutaping should be successful.

If you do not show any improvement after treatment with acutaping, there can be several reasons. The tape could be attached improperly. To check, the technique of taping should be compared with the illustrations in Part 2: How To Use Acutape. The different colors of the tape can be a problem as well. One patient might experience the blue tape as effective and comfortable, whereas another patient might experience it as uncomfortable and ineffective. Here, it is important to test for reactions first.

A Sightseeing Tour around the Human Body

The names of the bones and muscles that are used in this book will not always be familiar. This little "sightseeing tour" should help give you a better picture of the human body.

In Part 2: How To Use Acutape, the illustrations demonstrate the different procedures for self-treatment with acutaping. In these illustrations you can clearly make out the areas of the body that are being taped. However, to give you an even better understanding of the taping procedures, we are going to take a little tour through the human body's regions and structures—in other words, we will show you the anatomical landmarks.

Head, Chest, Abdominal, and Pelvic Regions

The trapezius muscle, a flat triangular muscle that covers the back of the neck, shoulders, and thorax, is prone to tension. It is attached at the base of the occipital bone at the back of the head, at the spinous process (a pointed outcropping) of the seventh cervical vertebra on the one side, and at the acromion process, a very strong bony ledge at the upper and outer side of the scapula (shoulder blade) on the other side. It is also attached to the spinous processes of all the thoracic vertebrae down to the twelfth thoracic vertebra, where, if you lie on your stomach, the smallest spinous process sticks up. The spinous processes of the vertebra run down the furrow of the back.

On the front side of the body below the neck, you can easily feel the breastbone and the ribs. The rib cage runs down close to the navel and separates the thorax from the abdomen. The lower abdomen is held in place by the strong pelvic bone (the ilium). The pelvic bone consists of two parts that are connected at the front of the body by a joint called the pubic symphysis. The joint between the sacrum (the triangular bone at the base of the spine) and the ilium is commonly known as the sacroiliac joint. The comfort of the lower back and the whole pelvic region relies heavily on the proper alignment of this joint. It is the central division between the spine, the pelvis, and the legs. Minor disorders of the leg joints and of organs in the pelvic area—such as the bladder, the bowels, the uterus in women, and the prostate in men—can lead to functional disorders of the spine as well.

The Arms

The arms are connected across the shoulder blades (the scapulae), and are connected to the back by a muscle group that starts at the scapulae and passes across the ribcage to the joints in the shoulder area. You can very easily feel the scapula and its acromion process, a very strong bony ledge at the upper and outer side. It prevents the ball of the upper arm from slipping out of joint. The biceps muscle can be seen at the front side of the upper arm, from the shoulder to the elbow. It is a muscle that easily can be felt all the way across the back of the upper arm until it reaches the point where the elbow extensor muscle attaches to the ulna bone in the lower arm. You can feel the bony knob at the lower end of the humerus (upper arm bone) on the outer side of the elbow joint. This is where the forearm and finger *extensor* muscle starts. The forearm and finger *flexor* muscle starts at the bony knob of the humerus on the inner side of the elbow joint. The styloid process of the ulna can be easily felt at the inner side of the wrist and at the outer side of the radius bone in the arm.

The Legs

At the outer side of the hip joint, the greater trochanter, a large knob at the top of the femur bone in the upper leg, can be easily felt. On the

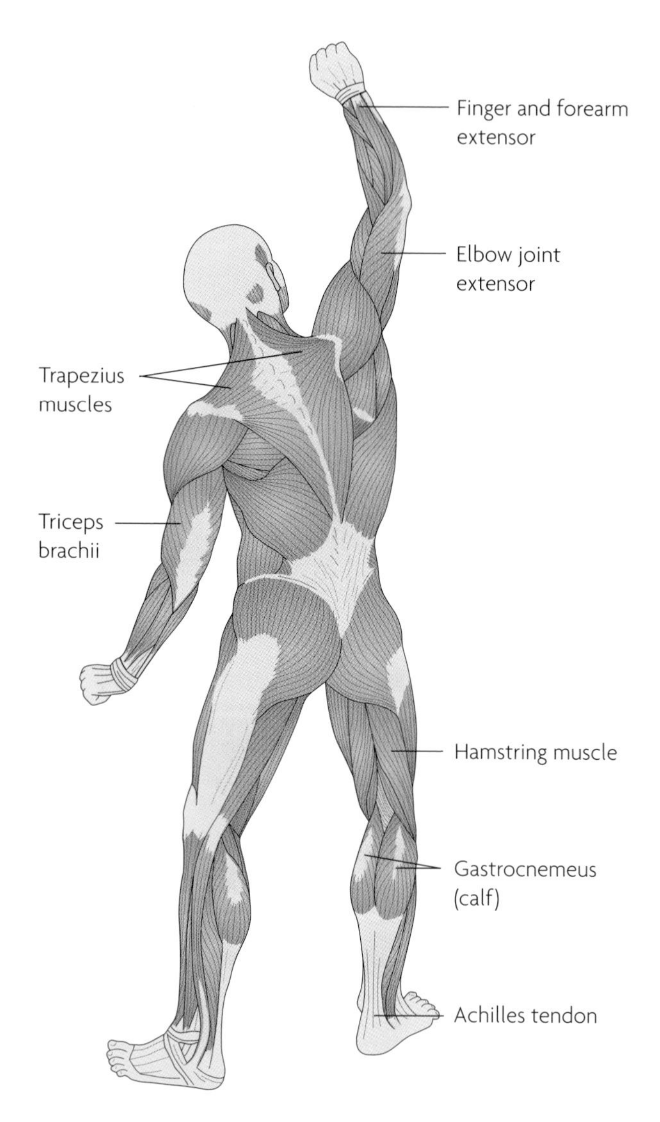

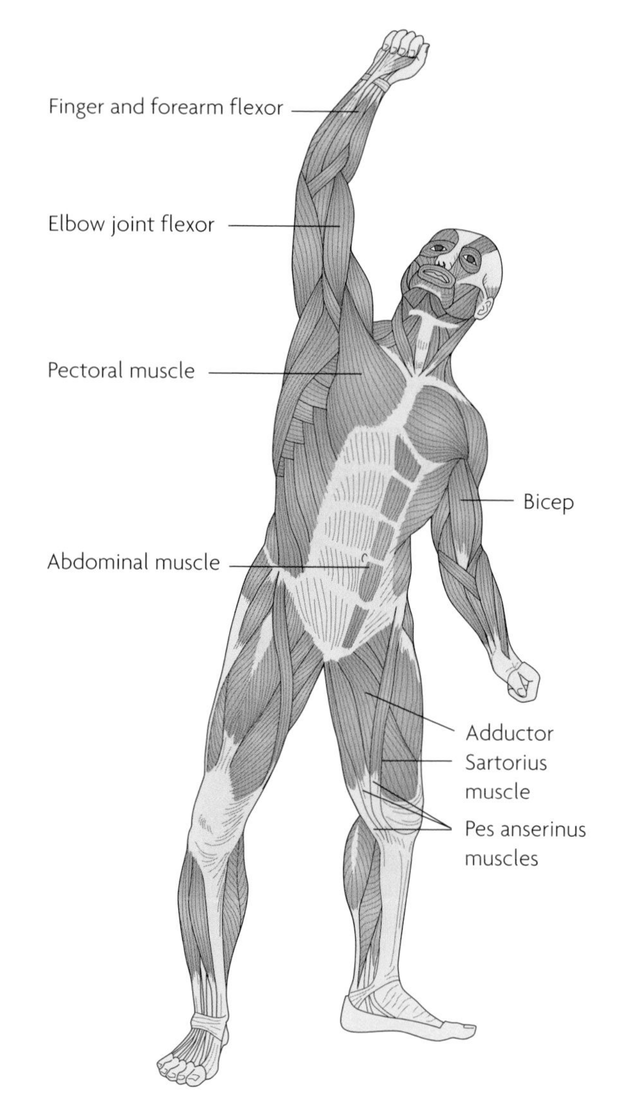

The human muscular system

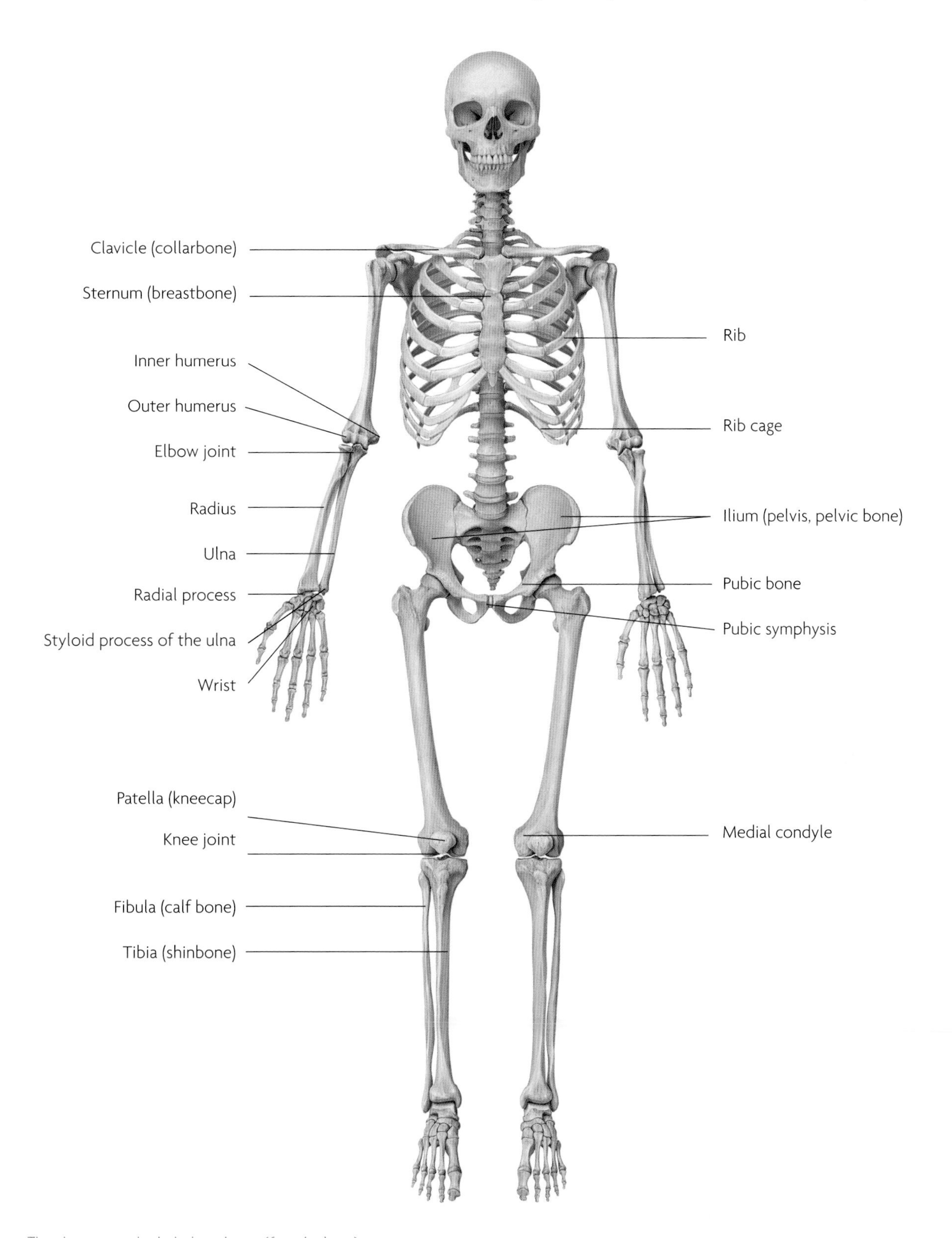

The human skeletal system (front view)

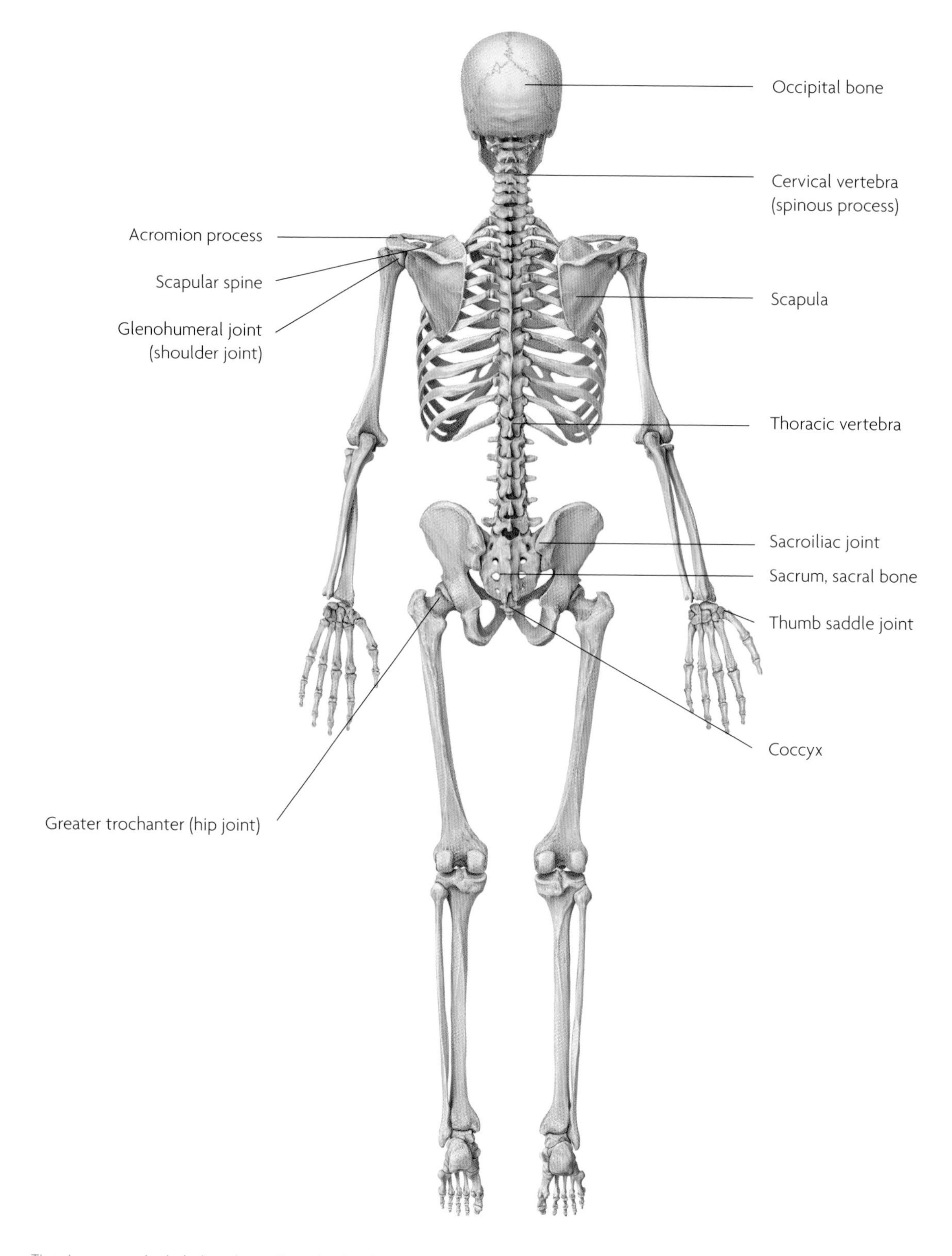

The human skeletal system (back view)

outer side of the knee joint you can feel the bony process at the lower end of the femur called the lateral condyle. On the inner side of the knee joint you can feel the medial condyle of the femur. The kneecap, which acts as a stabilizer, glides between them. The sartorius muscle is a long thigh muscle that starts at the lower part of the iliac crest and connects to a bony ledge at the outer part of the head of the shinbone, where the adductor muscles are also attached (these muscles are used to move the leg toward the body). The abductor muscles (with which we can move the leg sideways away from the body) are located between the pelvic bone and the greater trochanter of the femur in the hip joint.

The lower leg runs from the knee joint to the ankle joint. At the outer side of the knee joint you can feel the little head of the fibula (the smaller of the two lower leg bones), which extends a little into the hollow of the knee.

At the outer side of the lower leg between the shinbone (tibia) and the fibula, you find the muscles that move the foot toward the knee. At the back of the lower leg are the calf muscles; with those we move the foot away from the knee. At the inner side of the ankle joint you find the malleolus medialis; at the outer side, you find the distal fibula. Right before the heel bone you can feel the strong Achilles tendon.

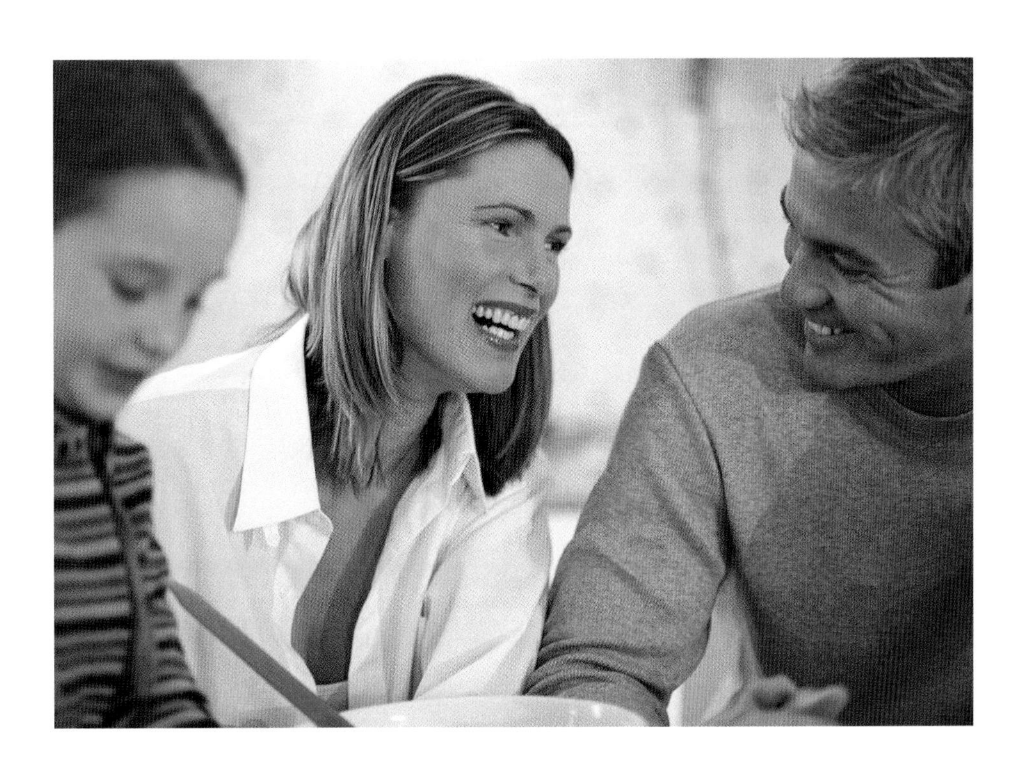

Part 2

HOW TO USE ACUTAPE

In the second part of the book we want to show you how to use acutape. Accompanying each description of how to use the tape in this section, you will find a list of all the ailments that can be treated effectively with it. Precise explanations as to how to attach the tape and other valuable tips and advice will help you gain confidence in using acutape very quickly. You will notice one thing early on: Acutaping is not difficult—and it is fun! The most important thing, of course, is that it is effective against so many disorders!

1. Finger and Forearm Extensor Tape

Ailments

- Pain in the area of the wrist
- Carpal tunnel syndrome (numbness in the area of the hand)
- Pain in the area of the elbow
- Tennis elbow
- Tendosynovitis (inflammation of the fluid-filled sheath surrounding a tendon)

Number and Length of Tapes

Number of Tapes: 2

Measuring the Tape

- **First strip of tape:** Runs from the back of the hand over the part of the forearm that faces out from the body, ending just above the outer elbow (2).
- **Second strip of tape:** Runs from the outer elbow around and over the part of the arm that faces toward the body, then down to the inner elbow (3).

Tip: Warm-up and stretch the muscles and joints so that the needed length of the tape can be measured exactly.

Preliminary Stretching and Attachment of the Tape

Preliminary Stretching

- Straighten your elbow and bend your wrist as far as possible to move the palm of your hand in the direction of the forearm (1). Then rotate your scooped hand from the wrist in the direction of the little finger (2).

Attaching the Tape

- The first strip of tape is attached first on the back of the hand, then up the forearm toward the side of the elbow facing away from the body, to just above the outer elbow itself (2).
- The second strip of tape is attached from the outer elbow inward toward the body and then it is angled down to the middle of the elbow (3).

Please Note

- You should stretch the strip of tape as little as possible while attaching it.
- The first strip of tape covers (on the back of your hand) the outer side of the wrist.

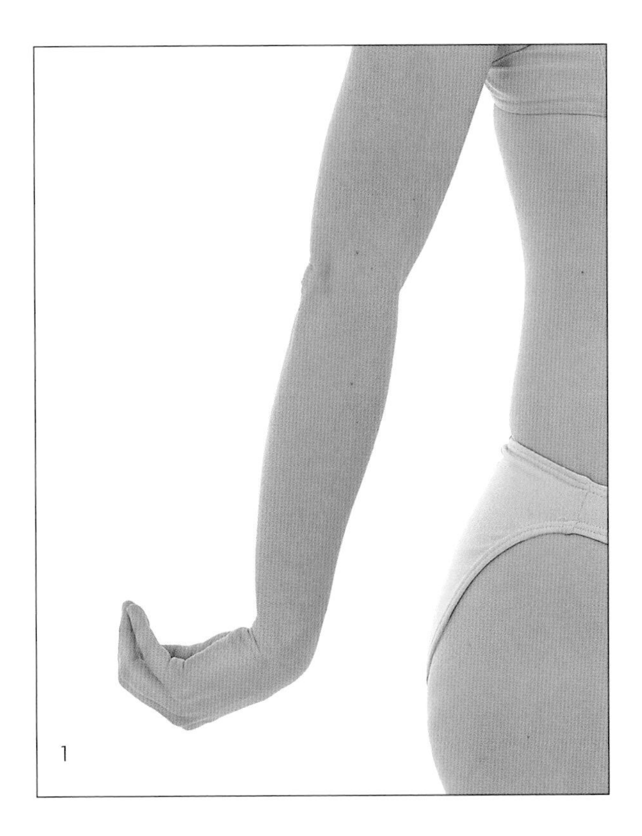

1

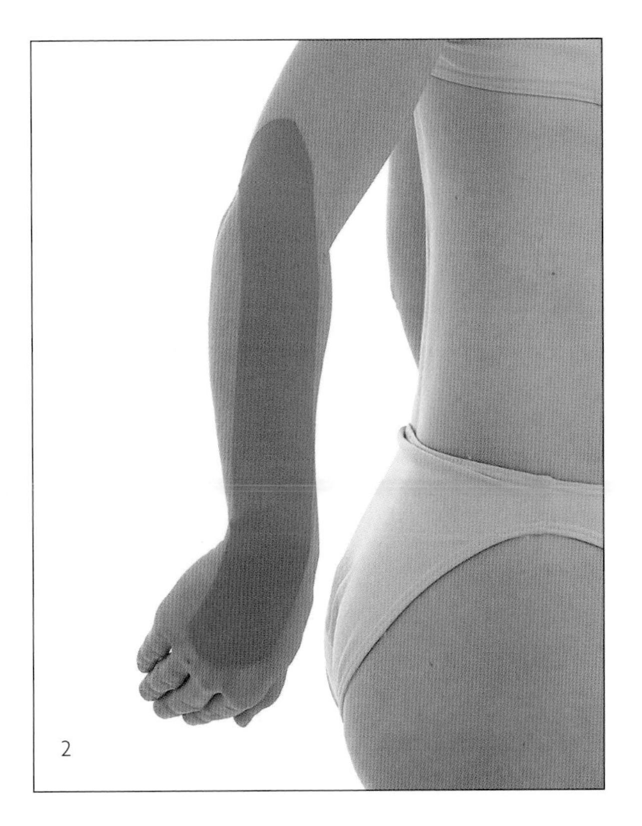

2

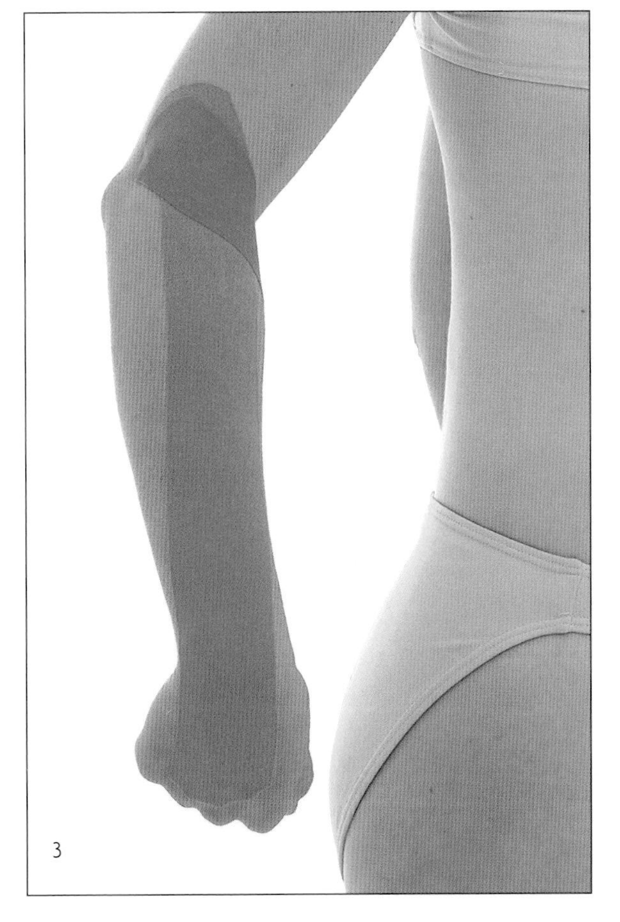

3

2. Finger and Forearm Flexor Tape

Ailments

- Pain in the area of the wrist
- Carpal tunnel syndrome (numbness in the area of the hand)
- Pain in the area of the elbow
- Golfer's elbow
- Tennis elbow
- Tendonitis (inflammation of a tendon)
- Vomiting (nausea) during pregnancy

Number and Length of Tapes

Number of Tapes: 3

Measuring the Tape

- **First strip of tape:** Runs from the middle of the palm of the hand over the inner side of the forearm to the part of the elbow that faces the body (3).
- **Second strip of tape:** Start it a little below the elbow joint at the outer side of the forearm and angle it up over the inner side of the elbow joint to end at the part of the elbow joint facing the body (4).
- **Third strip of tape:** Place it across the inner side of the wrist (4).

Tip: Do a preliminary stretching of the muscles and joints so you can measure the length of the tape strips exactly.

Preliminary Stretching and Attachment of the Tape

Preliminary Stretching

- Extend your arm straight from the elbow and lift your hand up (bending it at the wrist) as far as you can (1). Turn your forearm (at the elbow joint) to the outside in the direction of the little finger (2).

Attaching the Tape

- The first strip of tape is attached from the middle of the palm of the hand, over the part of the forearm that is facing the body, and further on over the side of the elbow facing the body (3).
- The second strip of tape is attached a little below the elbow joint at the part of the forearm facing away from the body, at an angle up to the inner side elbow joint, and over the side of the outer elbow joint facing the body (4).
- The third tape strip runs across the inner side of the wrist (4).

Please Note

- The tape covers the "funny bone" (actually a bundle of nerves), which is the sensitive spot that can be felt where the elbow faces the body.

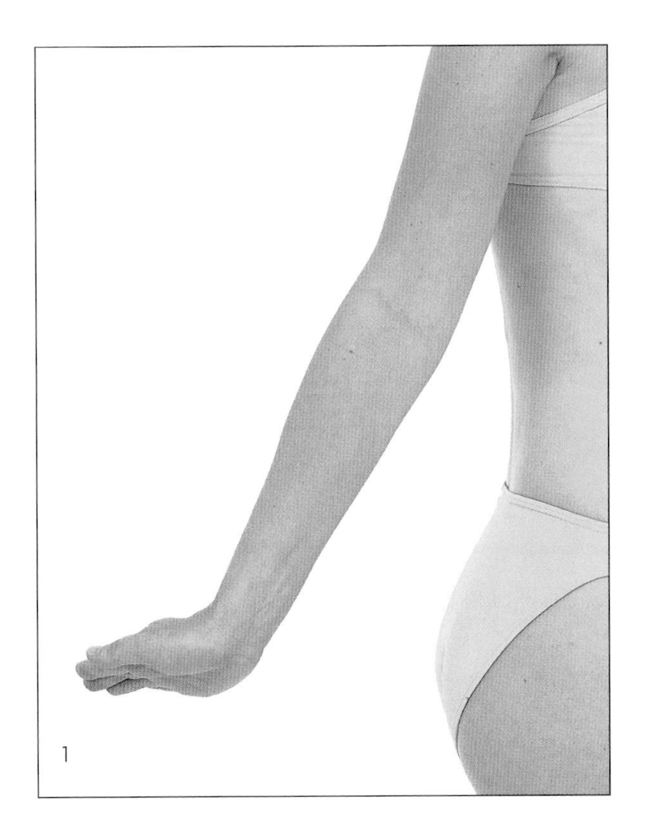
1

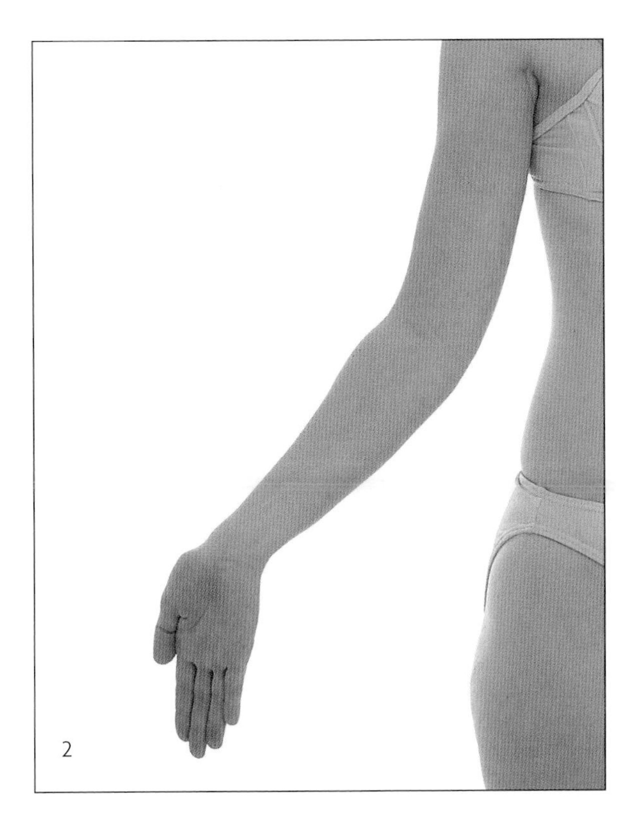
2

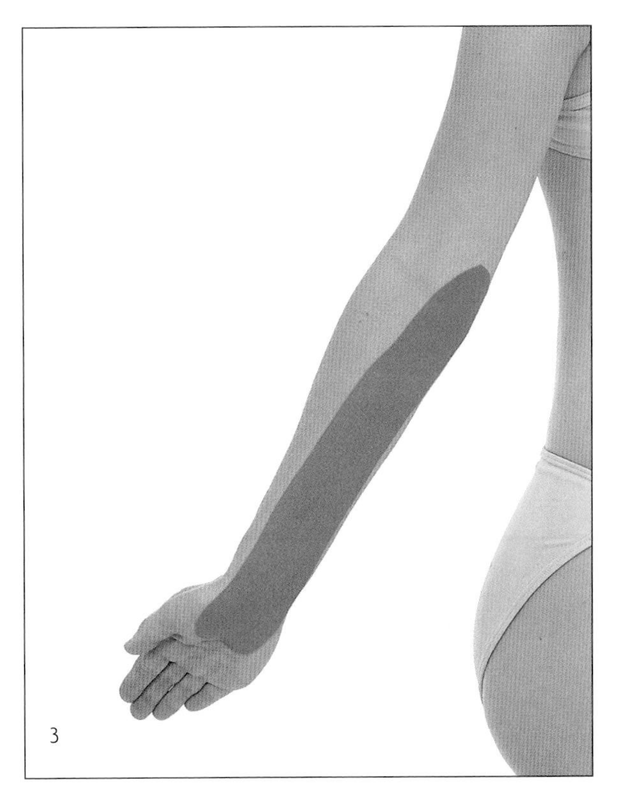
3

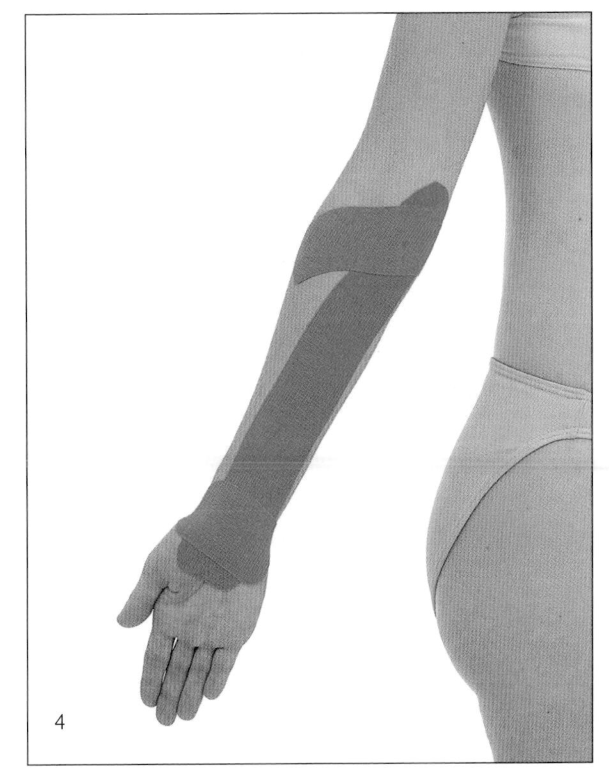
4

3. Thumb Saddle Joint Tape

Ailments

- Pain in the area of the thumb saddle joint
- Pain in the area of the wrist
- Carpal tunnel syndrome (numbness in the area of the hand)
- Tendonitis

Number and Length of Tapes

Number of Tapes: 2

Measuring the Tape

- **First strip of tape:** Runs from slightly above the thumb saddle joint straight up the forearm to just below the elbow (3).
- **Second strip of tape:** Crosses over the thumb saddle joint and over the inner palm of the hand so that the ball of the thumb is covered (4).

Tip: You can find the thumb saddle joint by using a finger to feel the spot between the base of the thumb and the middle of the inner wrist. This is where the thumb saddle joint is located. It is the joint that enables the thumb to move in a circle.

Preliminary Stretching and Attachment of the Tape

Preliminary Stretching

- Extend your arm at the elbow, your hand at the wrist, and your fingers so that they all are in a straight line. Turn the palm of your hand to face forward and bend the hand (at the wrist) in toward your body (1). Hold your thumb against the side of the forefinger and then bend it underneath the bottom side of the forefinger (2).

Attaching the Tape

- The first strip of tape is attached over the thumb saddle joint, goes straight up along the forearm, and ends just below the elbow (3).
- The second strip is taped across the thumb saddle joint (toward the palm of the hand) and over the ball of the thumb (4).

Please Note

- The thumb saddle joint has to be completely covered by the tape.

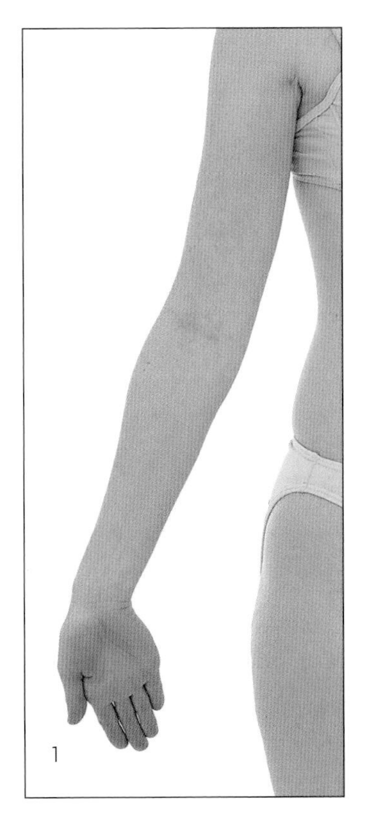
1

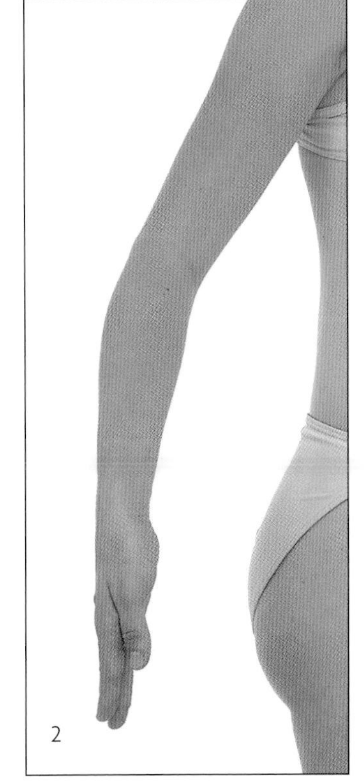
2

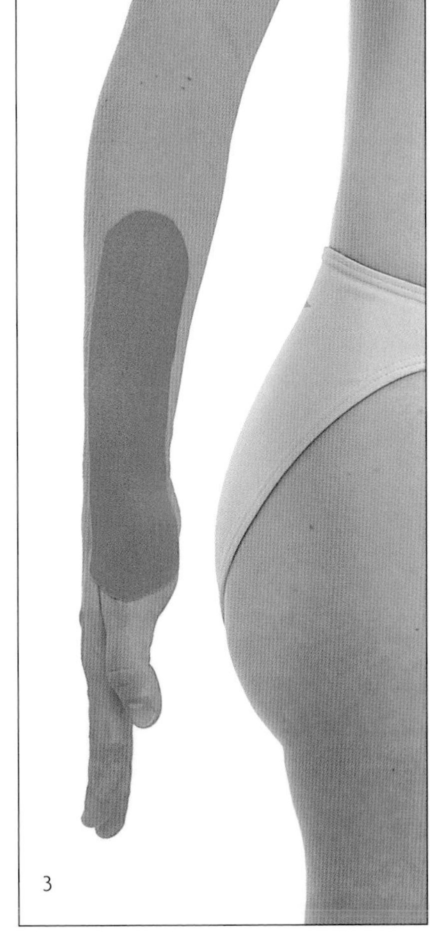
3

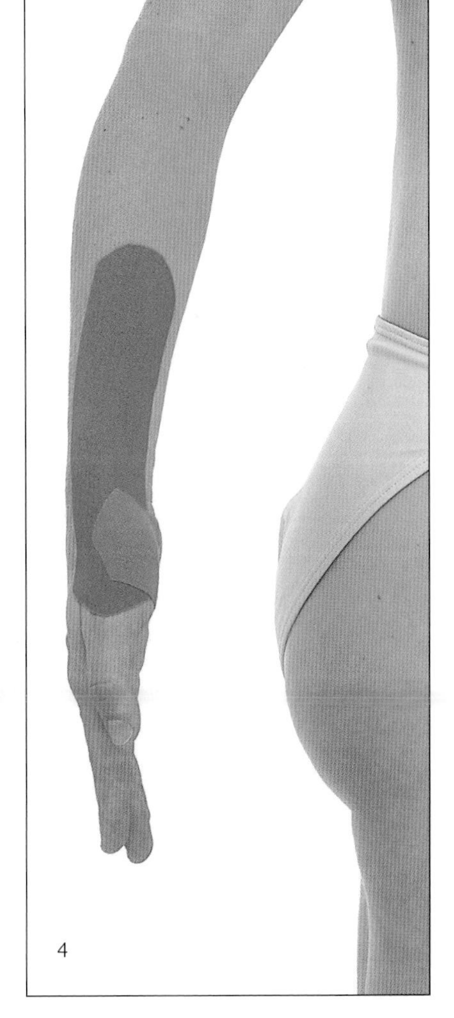
4

4. Elbow Joint Extensor Tape

Ailments

- Pain in the area of the shoulder
- Pain in the area of the elbow
- Tennis elbow
- Golfer's elbow
- Back pain in the area of the cervical, thoracic, and lumbar portions of the spine

Number and Length of Tapes

Number of Tapes: 1

Measuring the Tape

- The tape runs from the lower part of the scapula to the point of the elbow (2).

Tip: Do a preliminary stretch of the muscles and joints so you can measure the length of the tape strip exactly.

Preliminary Stretching and Attachment of the Tape

Preliminary Stretching

- Bend your arm at the elbow joint as much as possible and raise it up so that you can reach back and touch the scapula with the palm of your hand (1).

Attaching the Tape

- The tape strip is attached from the lower part of the scapula, along the back of the upper arm, and over the point of the elbow (2).

Please Note

- You should do the preliminary stretching of your upper arm and the shoulder area as thoroughly as possible.

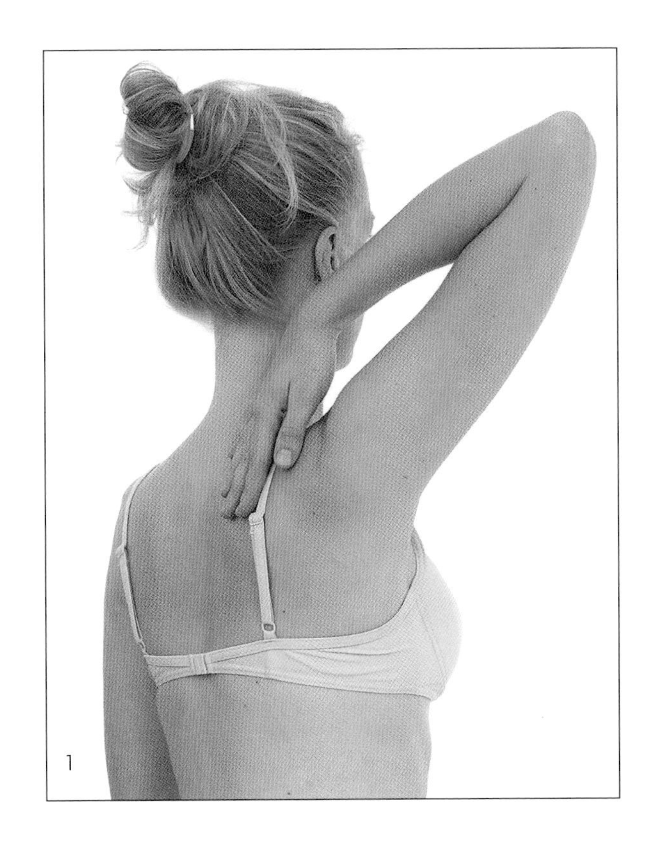

1

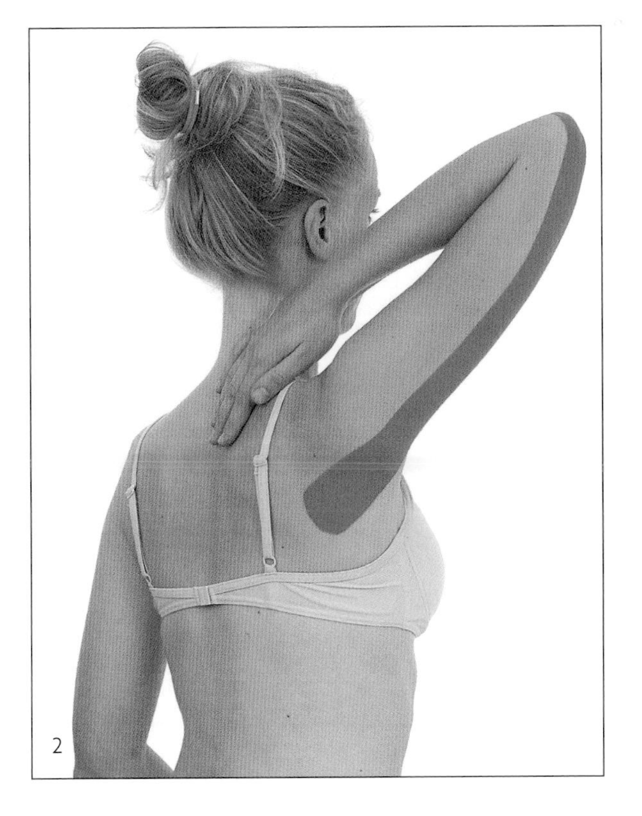

2

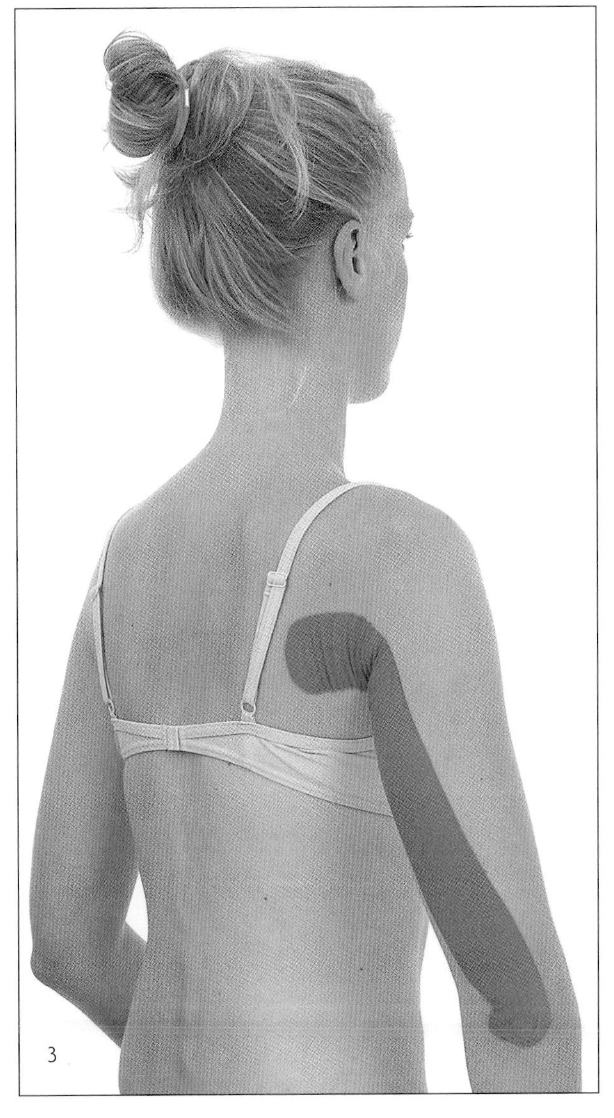

3

5. Elbow Joint Flexor Tape

Ailments

- Pain in the area of the elbow
- Tennis elbow
- Pain in the area of the upper arm
- Pain in the area of the shoulder

Number and Length of Tapes

Number of Tapes: 1

Measuring the Tape

- The tape runs along the inner side of the forearm starting slightly below the bend of the elbow, over the biceps, and up to the shoulder (2).

Tip: Do a preliminary stretching of the muscles and joints so you can measure the length of the tape strips exactly.

Important: The upper part of the tape should be positioned on the outer shoulder first, before attaching it, and then the top of the tape strip should be cut to down the middle so that each cut piece can be attached separately on the front of the shoulder (3)!

Preliminary Stretching and Attachment of the Tape

Preliminary Stretching

- Stretch your arm out straight and turn the palm of your hand toward the back, then move the whole arm to the back, pivoting it away from your body from the shoulder joint (1).

Attaching The Tape

- The end of the tape strip that is not split is positioned on the inner side of the forearm slightly below the elbow joint and is attached from there up to the front of the shoulder. In the area of the armpit, the split end of the tape is attached with one side of the split tape more toward the neck and the other side of the split tape more toward the shoulder joint (2).

Please Note

- The tape is attached starting on the forearm and then over the inner side of the elbow joint.

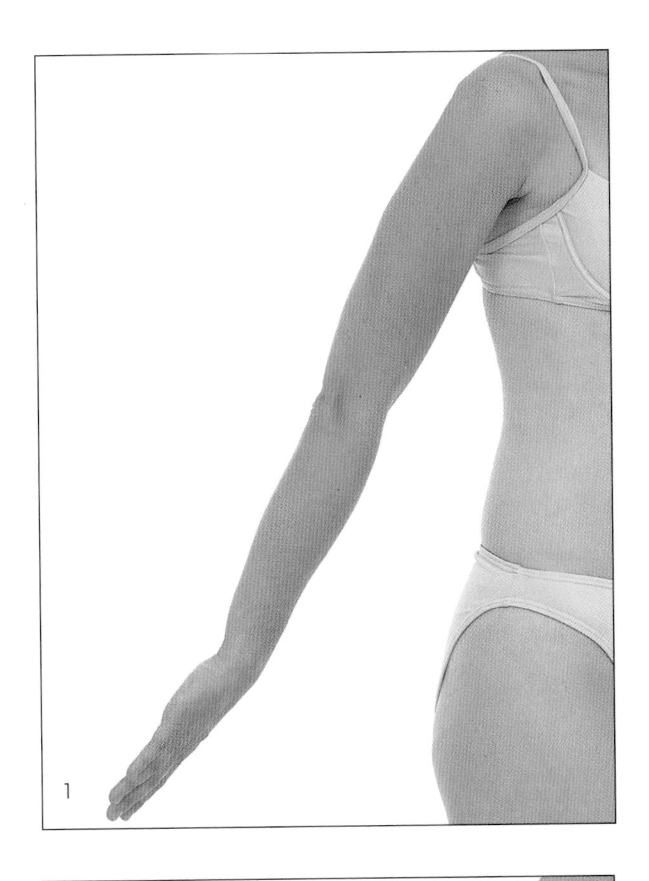

1

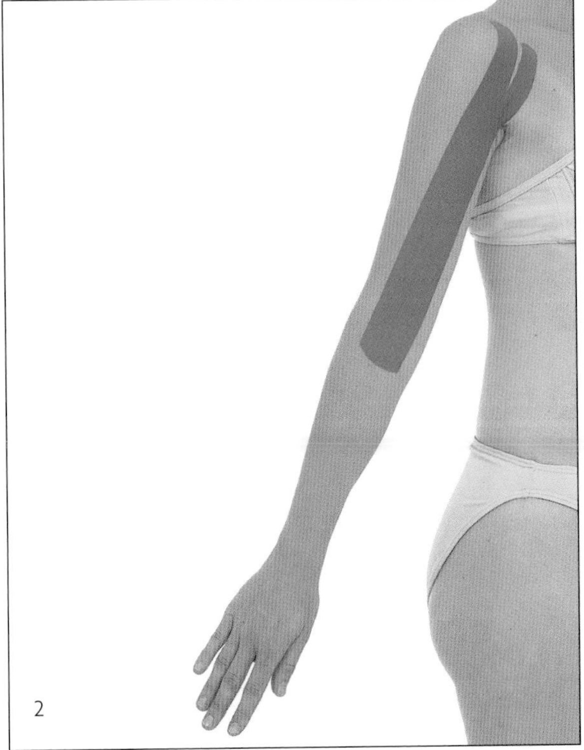

2

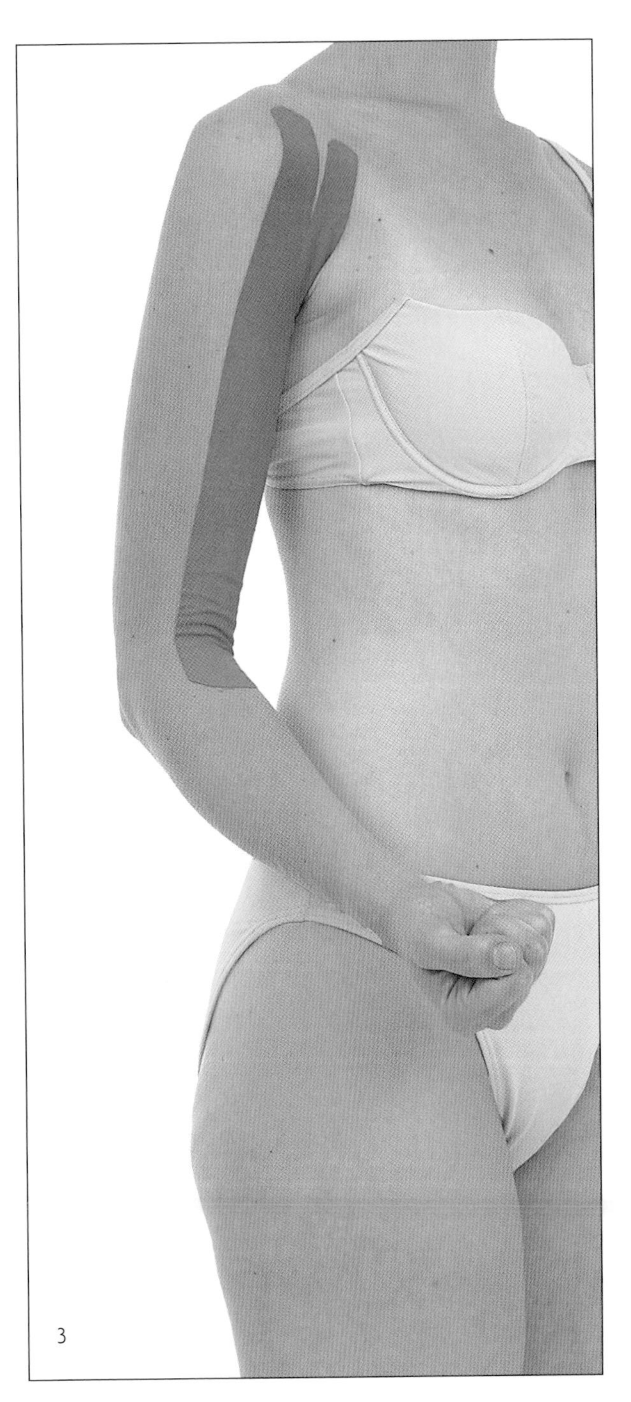

3

6. Pectoral Muscle Tape

Ailments

- Pain in the area of the shoulder
- Pain in the area of the rib cage

Number and Length of Tapes

Number of Tapes: 2

Measuring the Tape

- **First strip of tape:** Runs crosswise from the upper arm slightly below the shoulder joint to almost (but not quite) the middle of the chest (2).
- **Second strip of tape:** Runs crosswise from the upper arm, a little farther below the shoulder joint than the first tape, all the way to the middle of the breastbone (3).

Tip: Do a preliminary stretching of the muscles and joints so you can measure the length of the tape strips exactly.

Preliminary Stretching and Attachment of the Tape

Preliminary Stretching

- Lift your extended arm to shoulder height so that the arm is straight out from the body. Turn the palm of your hand to the front and bend the elbow joint so that the tips of your fingers point straight up (1).

Attaching the Tape

- The first strip of tape is attached at the upper arm a little below the shoulder; from there it is attached below the collarbone, running almost to the middle of the chest (2).
- The second strip starts a little lower on the upper arm and runs and all the way to the middle of the breastbone (3).

Please Note

- Except where it is specifically called for, we do not work with split tape but with two separate tapes. This taping protocol is more effective with two whole tapes when it reaches the pectoral muscle.

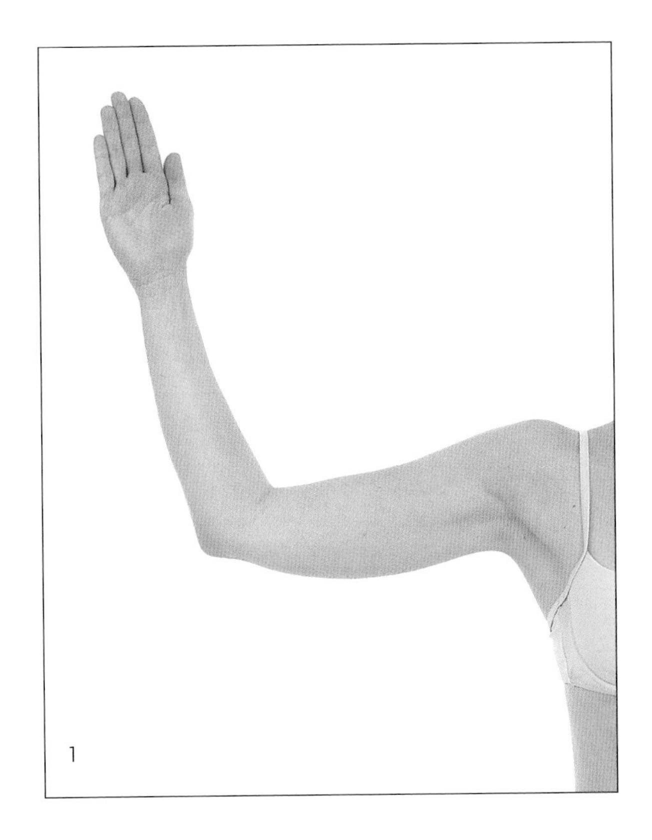

1

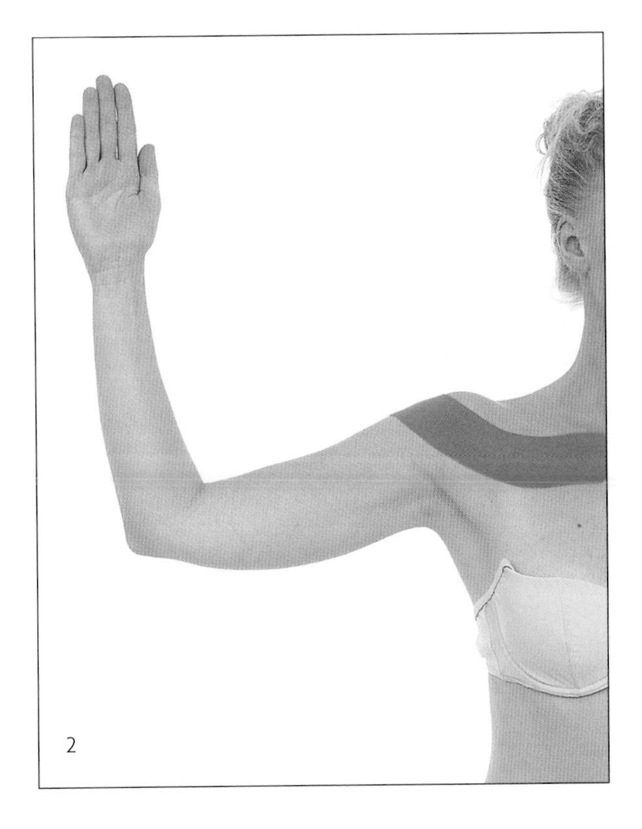

2

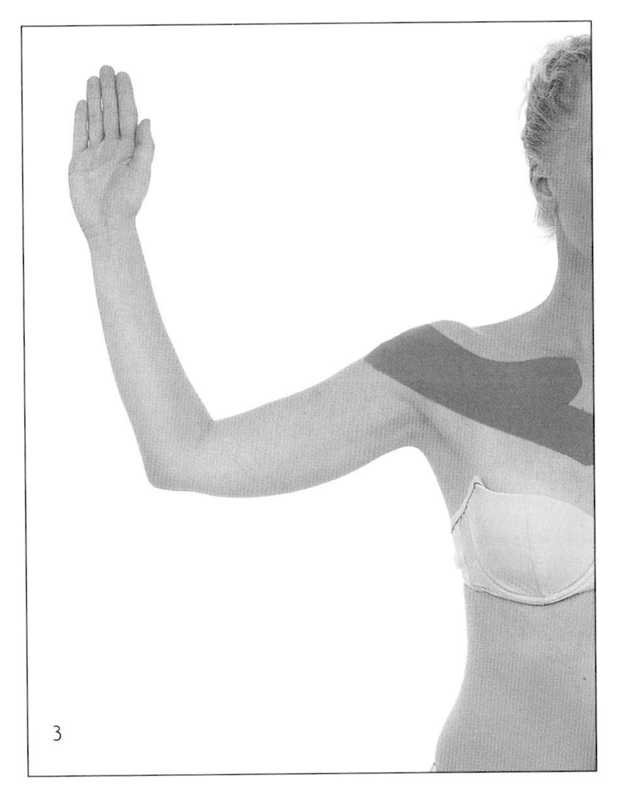

3

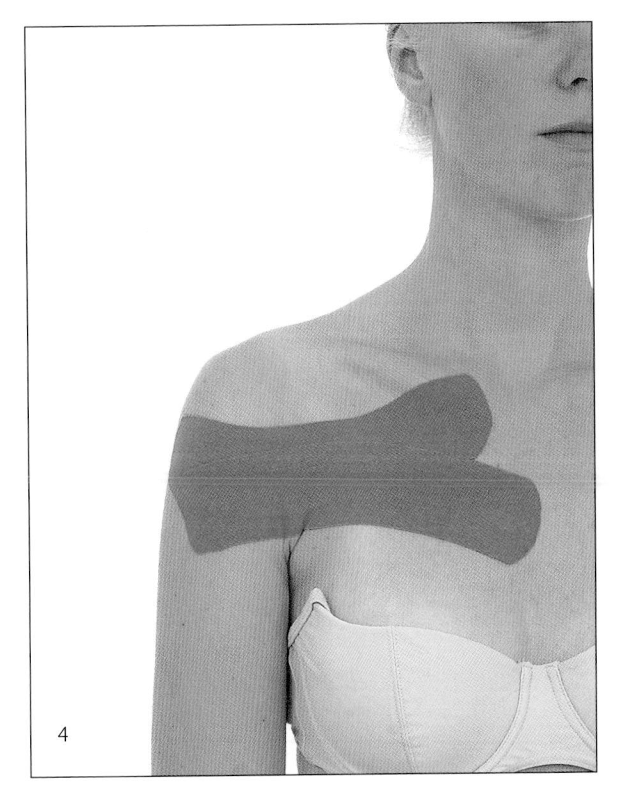

4

7. Trapezius Muscle Tape

Ailments

- Pain in the area of the shoulder
- Pain in the area of the cervical spine
- Headaches
- Dizziness
- Ringing in the ears (tinnitus)

Number and Length of Tapes

Number of Tapes: 3

Measuring the Tape

- **First strip of tape:** Looking at the body from the back, this tape runs from the hairline at the side of the neck, along the top of the shoulder, to the shoulder joint (2).
- **Second strip of tape:** Runs horizontally across the back from the thoracic spine, over the scapula, to the back of the shoulder joint (5).
- **Third strip of tape:** Begins at the transition point one third of the way up the back where the lumbar portion of the spine changes to the thoracic spine, and runs diagonally across the back to the back of the shoulder joint (8).

Tip: Do a preliminary stretching of the muscles and joints so you can measure the length of the tape strips exactly.

Preliminary Stretching and Attachment of the Tape

First Strip of Tape

- **Preliminary stretching:** Tilt your head slightly toward the side that is not being taped (1).
- **Attaching the tape:** Begin at the hairline at the side of the neck and run the tape along the top of the shoulder to the shoulder joint (2).

Second Strip of Tape

- **Preliminary stretching:** Move the arm that is on the side that is being taped, across the front of your body at shoulder height and hold on to opposite shoulder with your hand (3). With your free hand, gently pull down on the elbow of the arm that is crossing your body (4).

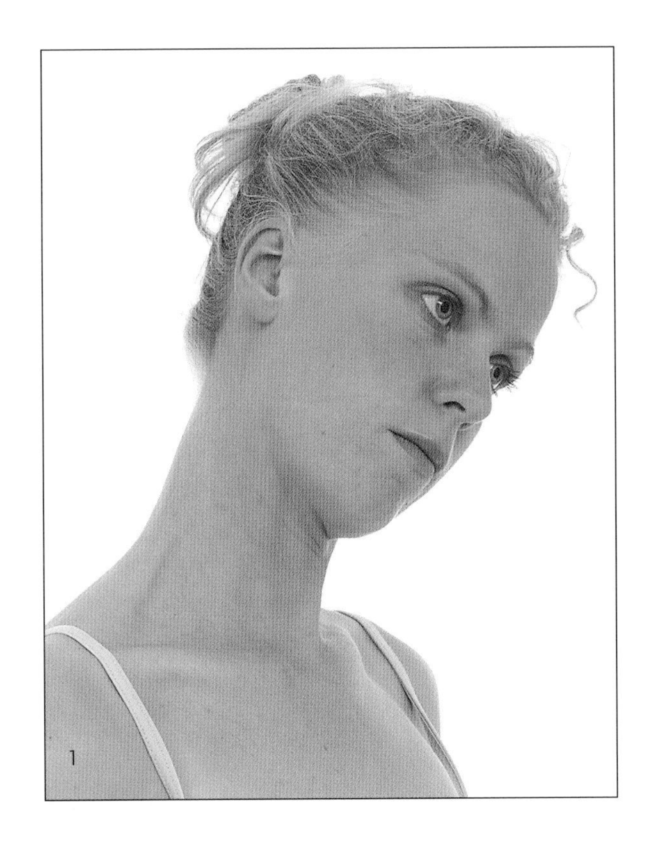
1

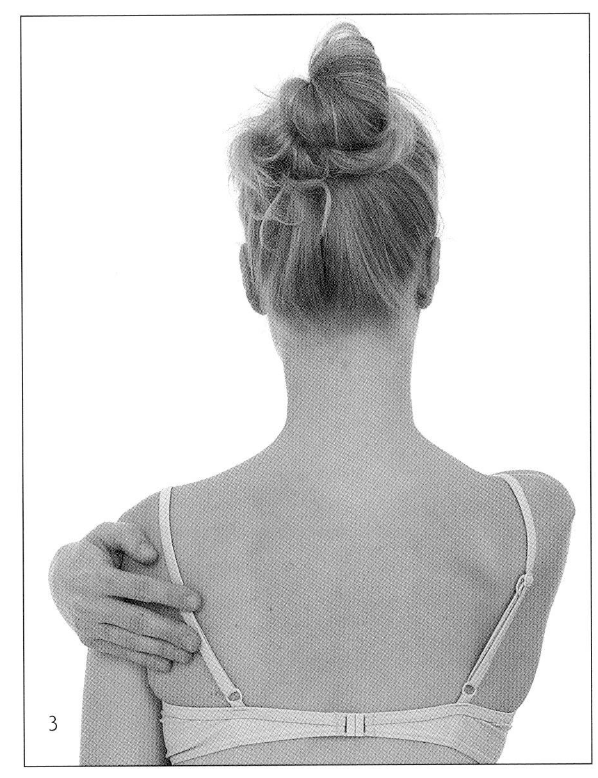
3

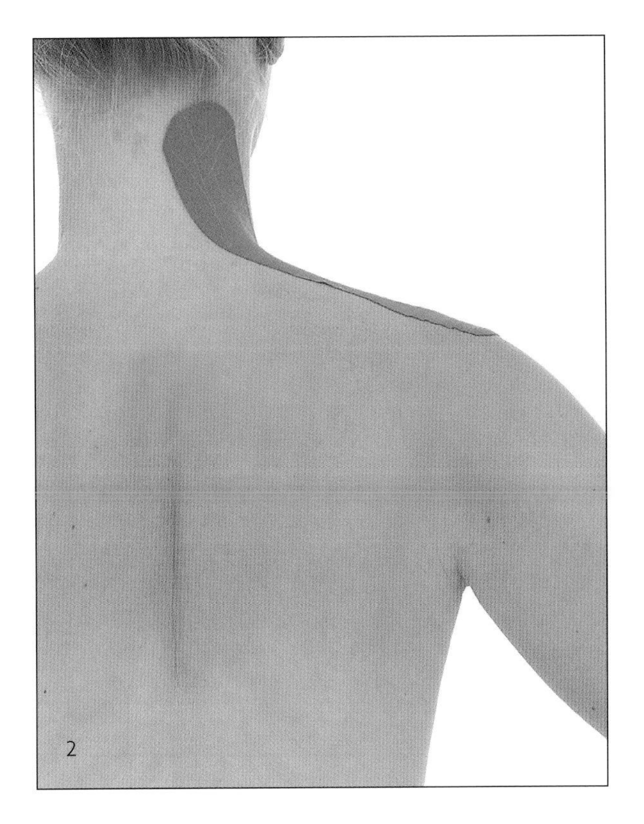
2

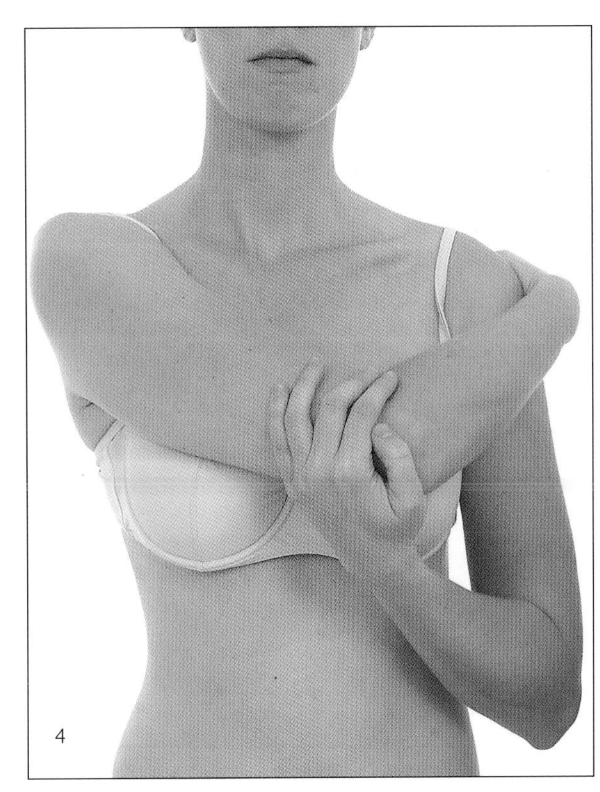
4

- **Attaching the tape:** Begin at the thoracic spine and attach the tape over the middle of the scapula to the back of the shoulder joint (5).

Third Strip of Tape

- **Preliminary stretching:** Place the palm of the hand on the side that is being taped on at the nape of the neck on that same side (6). Then tilt your head toward the other side (7).
- **Attaching the tape:** Begin on the spine at the transition point where the lumbar section of the spine changes to the thoracic spine and run the tape diagonally across the back to the back of the shoulder joint (8).

Please Note

- The trapezius muscle runs in two strands on either side of the spine from the shoulders all the way up the neck to the occipital bone.
- Therefore, this tape works very well in treating ailments of the nape of the neck and shoulders.

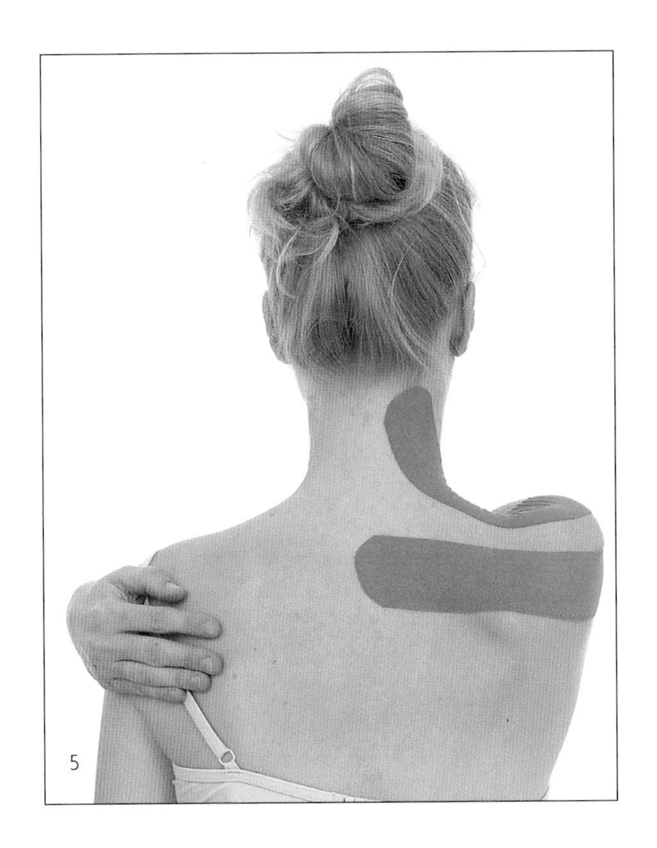
5

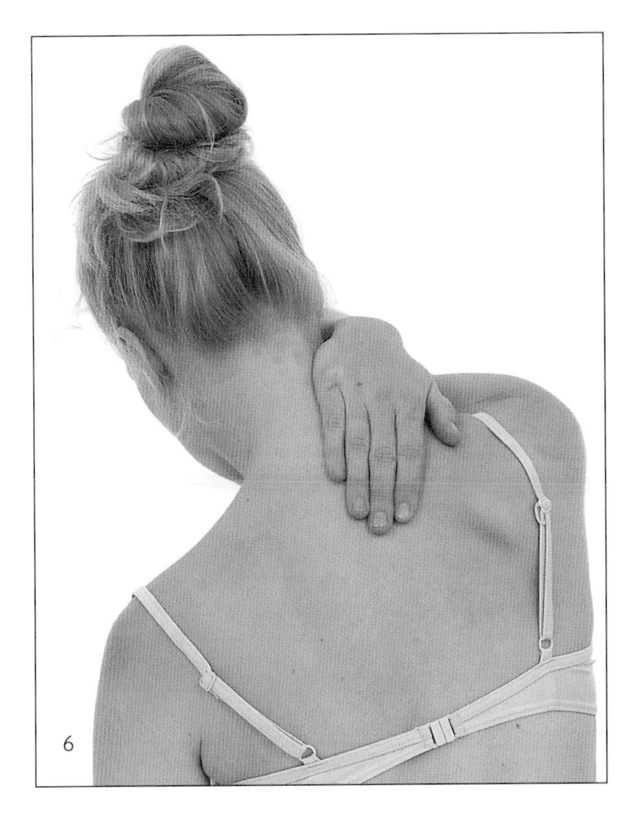
6

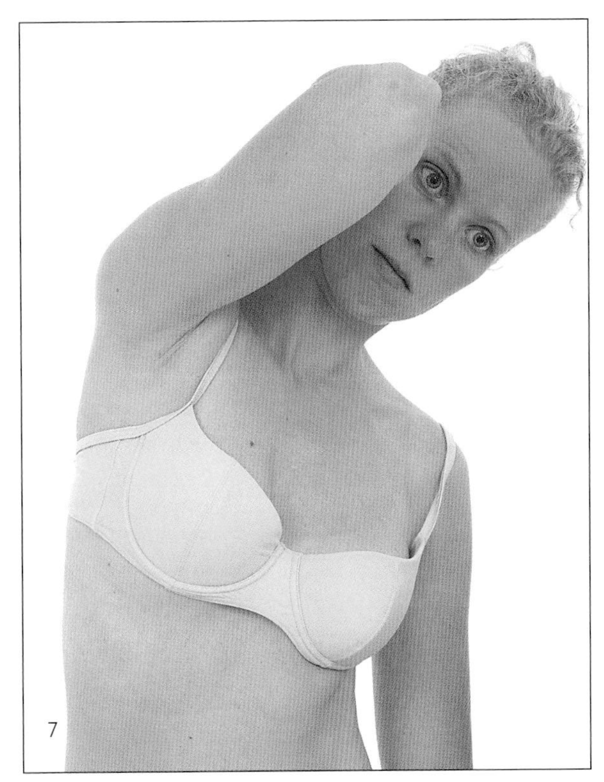
7

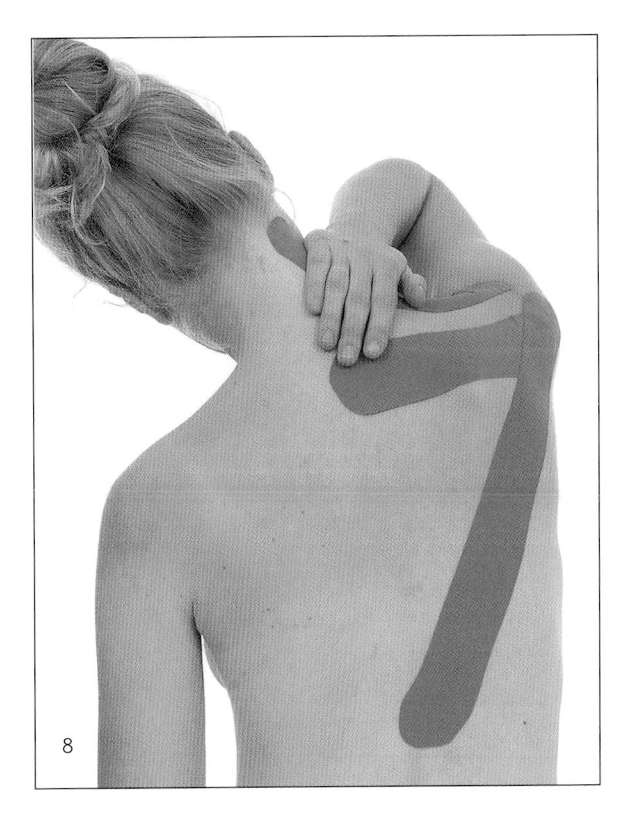
8

8. Levator Scapula Muscle Tape

Ailments

- Pain in the area of the shoulder
- Headache
- Pain in the area of the cervical spine
- Dizziness
- Ringing in the ears (tinnitus)

Number and Length of Tapes

Number of Tapes: 1

Measuring the Tape

- The tape runs from the hairline at the back of the neck, straight down over the scapula (2).

Tip: Do a preliminary stretching of the muscles and joints so you can measure the length of the tape strip exactly.

Preliminary Stretching and Attachment of the Tape

Preliminary Stretching

- Put your hand lightly against your head on the side that is being taped; tilt your head slightly to the other side and a little bit forward (1).

Attaching the Tape

- The strip of tape is attached from the hairline at the back of the neck straight down next to the spine and over the inner edge of the scapula (2).

Please Note

- You should do the preliminary stretch for this area exactly as it is described.
- The levator scapula muscle is affected by nearly all disorders found in the areas of the shoulder and the nape of the neck. It is important that the tape cover the whole length of the inner edge of the scapula along the spine.
- You can tape the levator scapulae on both sides of the spine at one time if necessary.

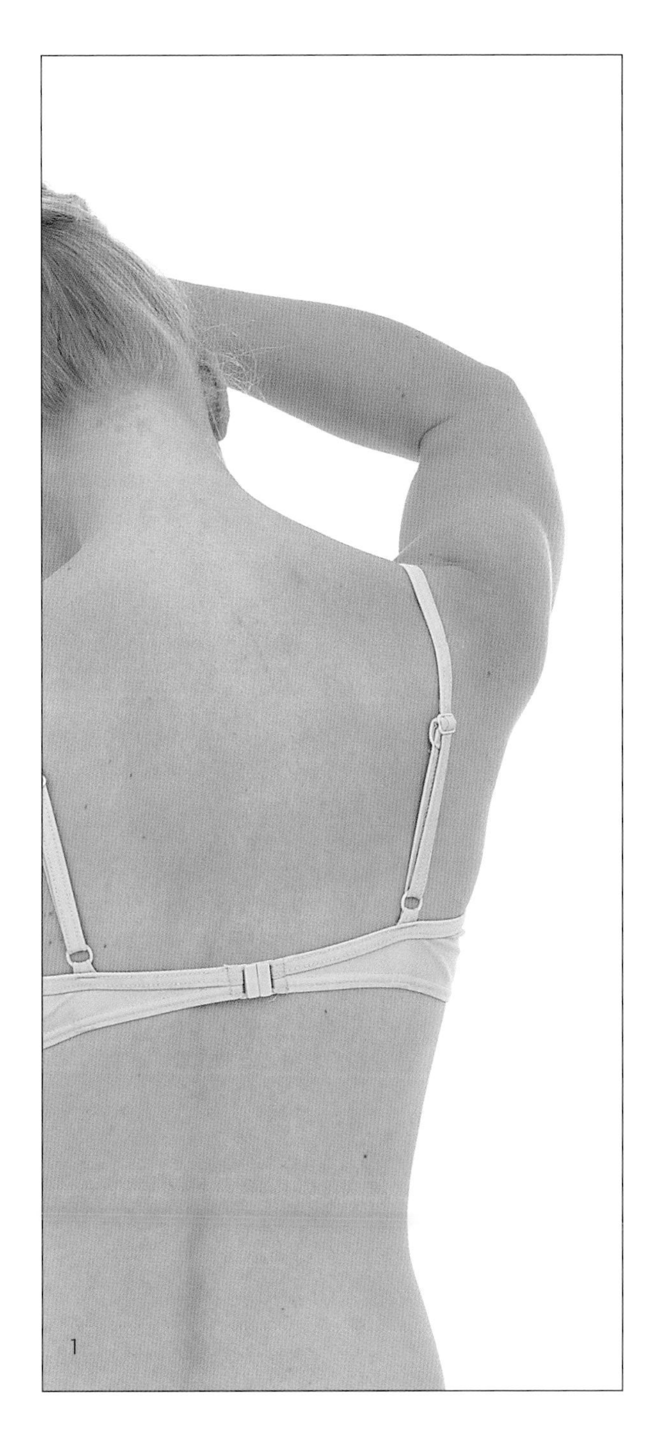
1

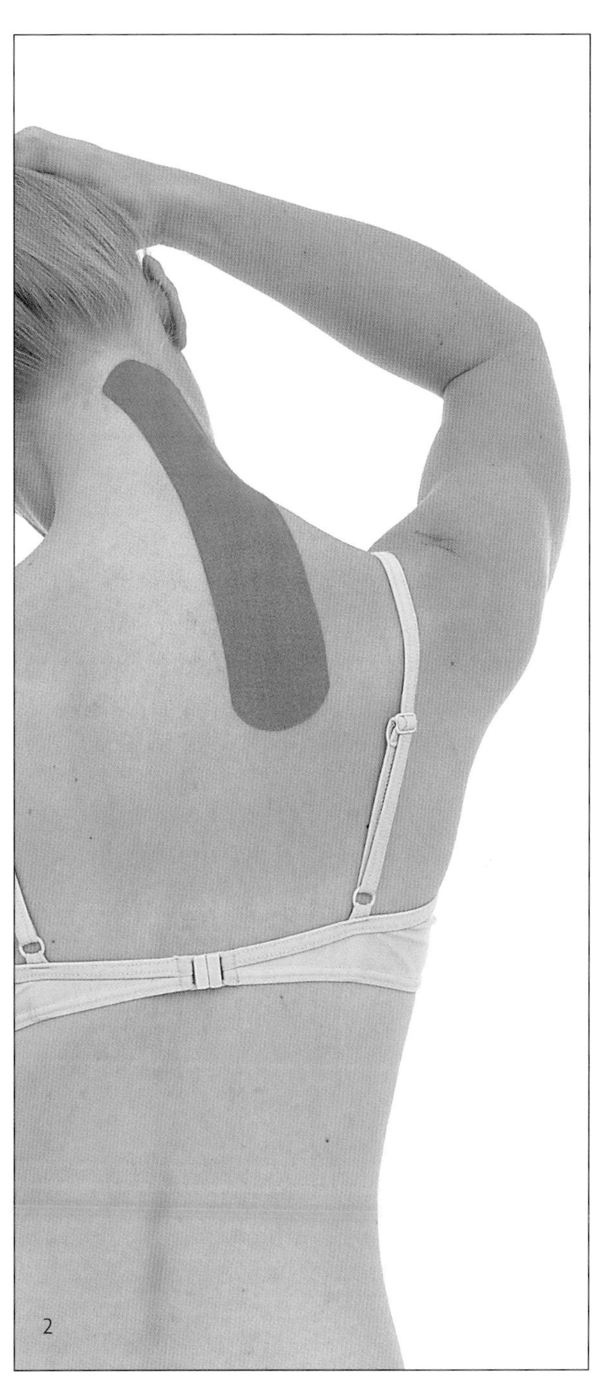
2

9. Rotator Cuff Muscle Tape

Ailments

- Pain in the area of the shoulder
- Pain in the area of the upper arm

Number and Length of Tapes

Number of Tapes: 2

Measuring the Tape

- **First strip of tape:** Begins at the base of the neck and runs over the shoulder, to the upper part of the arm (2).
- **Second strip of tape:** Runs horizontally across the whole scapula, to the upper arm (2).

Tip: Do a preliminary stretching of the muscles and joints so you can measure the length of the tape strips exactly.

Preliminary Stretching and Attachment of the Tape

Preliminary Stretching

- Put the arm (of the side that is being taped) behind your back with the forearm across the lumbar region of the spine and turn the palm of the hand out (1).

Attaching the Tape

- The first tape strip is attached from base of the neck along the top of the shoulder to the upper part of the arm (2).
- The second strip is attached from the middle of the inner edge of the scapula to the upper part of the arm (2).

Please Note

- It is all right if you find that you are not able to do the preliminary stretching of the shoulder and neck region as described. Remember that the degree of stretch is always a matter of individual capability. The tape can still be stretched before attaching.
- The rotator cuff muscle tape shown here consists of two tapes: one for the upper rotator cuff muscle and one for the lower rotator cuff muscle.

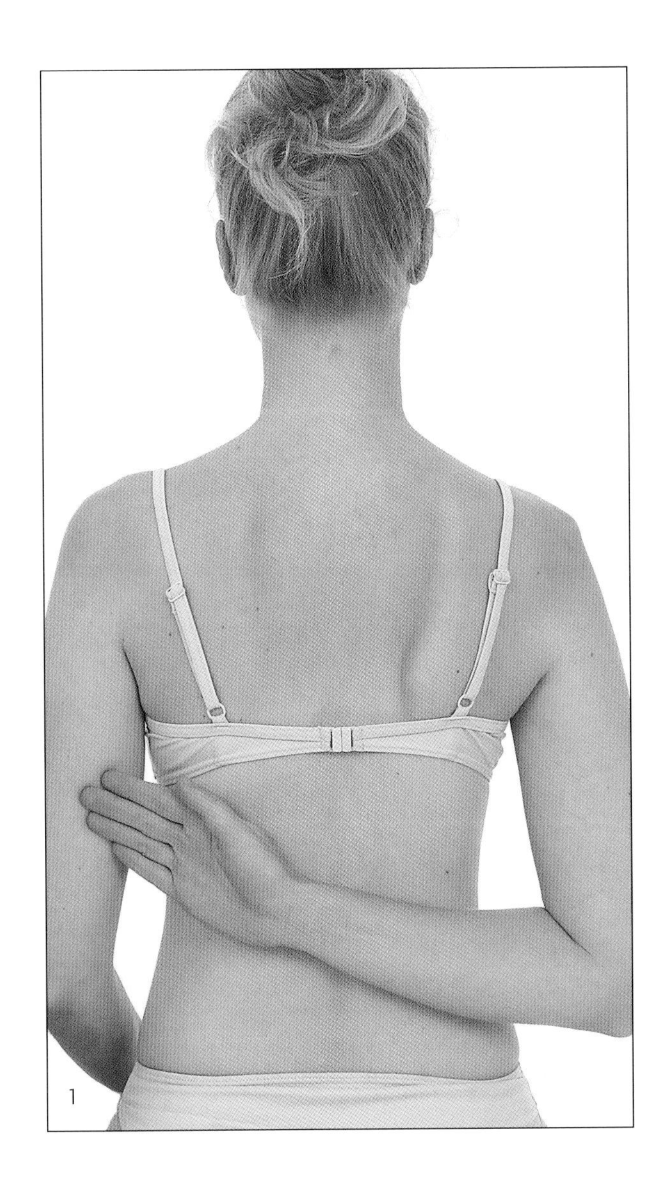
1

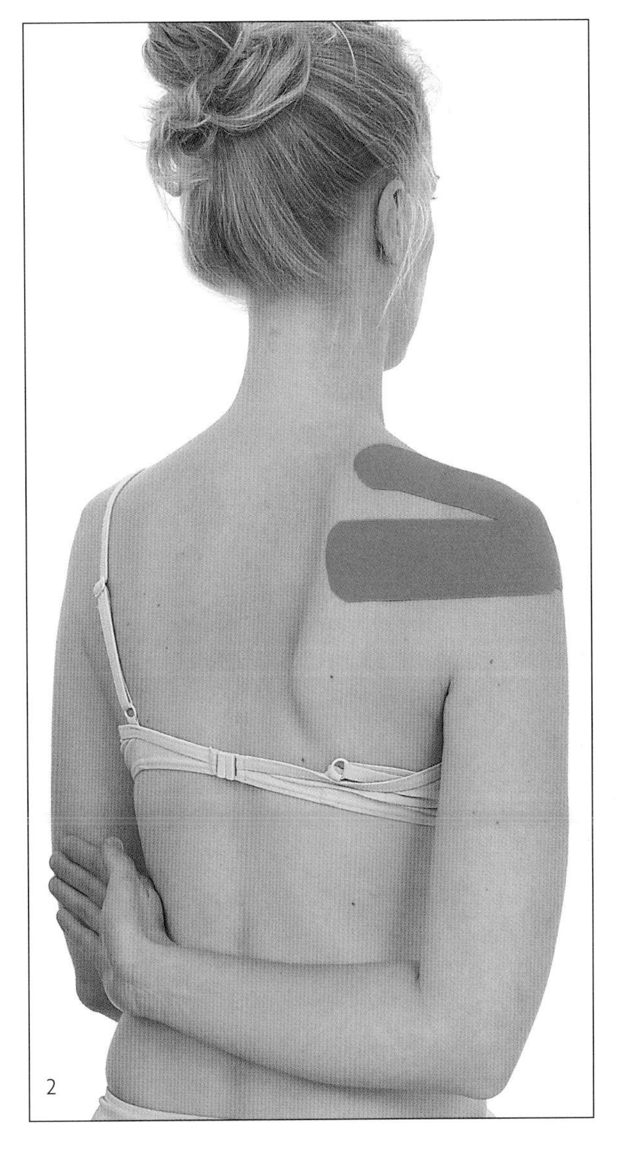
2

10. Levator Costarum (or Scalenus) Muscle Tape

Ailments

- Pain in the area of the upper arm
- Pain in the area of the shoulder
- Headaches
- Pain in the area of the cervical spine

Number and Length of Tapes

Number of Tapes: 1

Measuring the Tape

- The tape runs straight down the neck from the head, starting behind the ear, to slightly before the collarbone (2).

Tip: Do a preliminary stretching of the muscles and joints so you can measure the length of the tape strips exactly.

Important: Cut the tape strip into a cone shape.

Preliminary Stretching and Attachment of the Tape

Preliminary Stretching

- Tilt your head away from the side that is being taped (1).

Attaching the Tape

- Attach the smaller end of the tape strip behind the ear. From there the tape should run straight down the neck, with the wide end attached slightly above your collarbone (2).

Please Note

- The tape runs down the front side of your neck in the direction of the collarbone because there are trigger points there. Trigger points are sensitive points that can be painful themselves or can trigger pain in other areas of the body. Below the collarbone is the first rib. With the levator costarum muscle tape you also can treat these trigger points in the neck and any blockages in the area of the first rib.
- In medical terminology, this tape is also called scalenus tape, after the scalenus muscle of the neck.

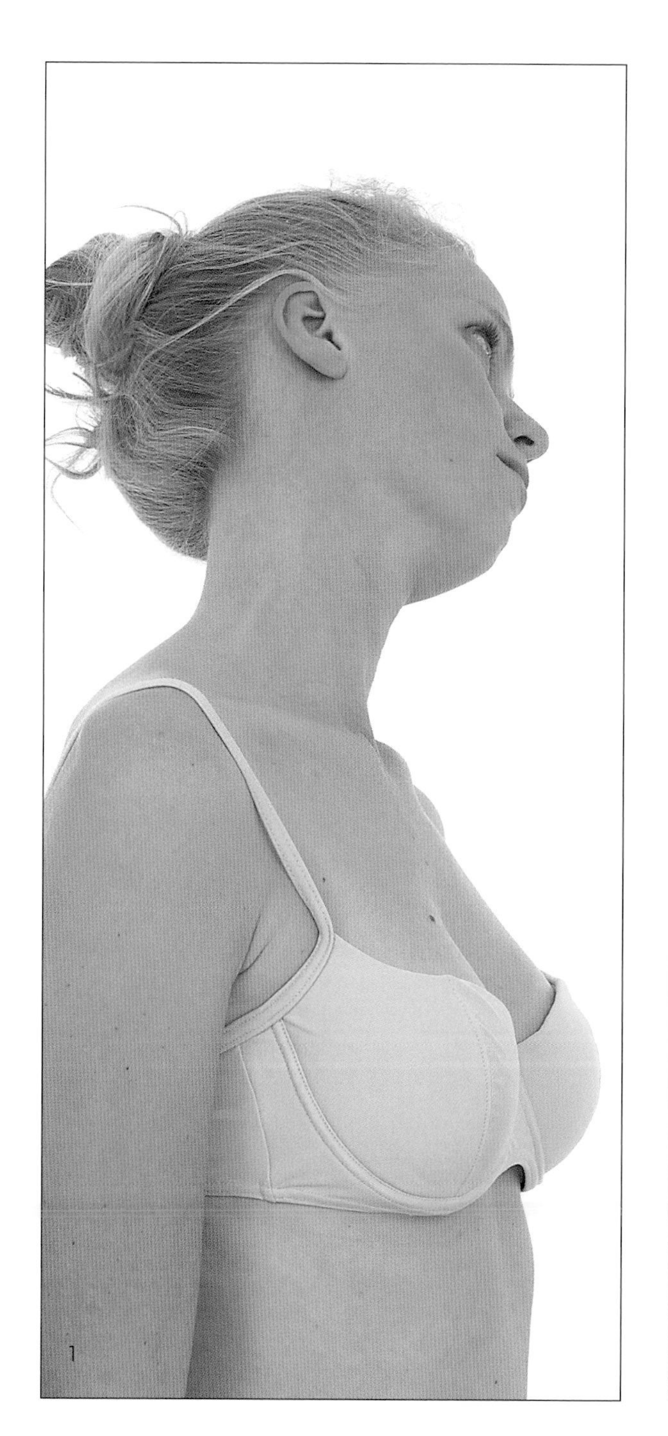

1

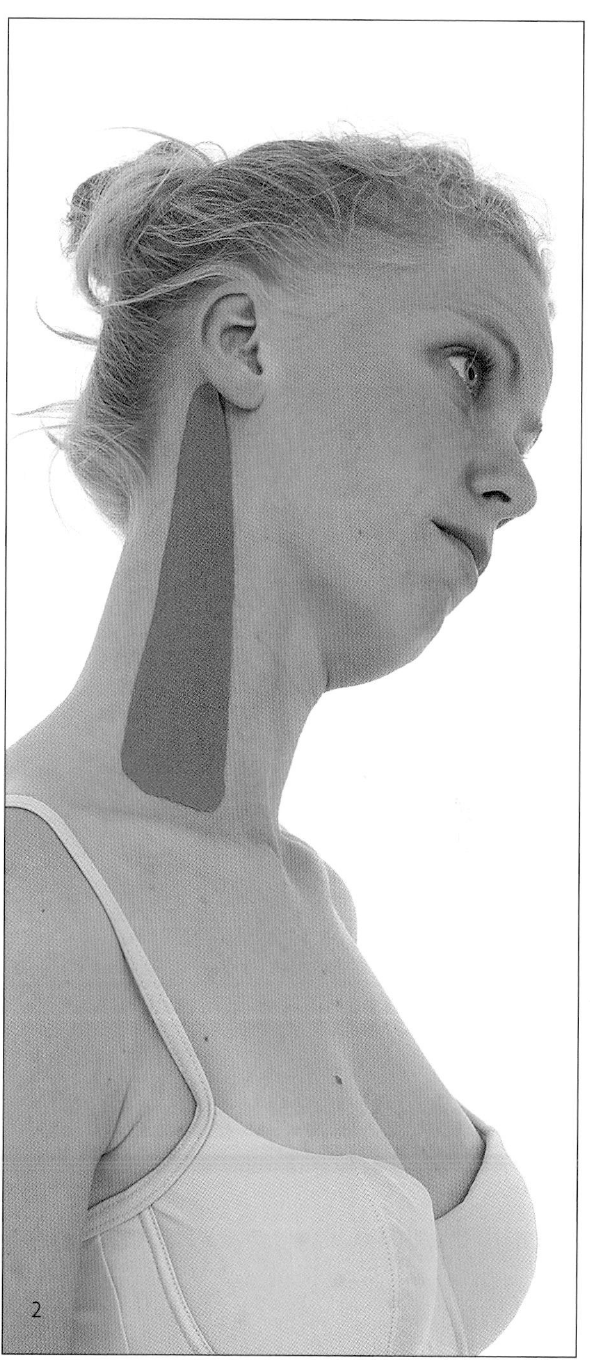

2

11. Rhomboid Muscle Tape

Ailments

- Pain in the area of the shoulder
- Pain in the area of the thoracic spine

Number and Length of Tapes

Number of Tapes: 2

Measuring the Tape

- **First strip of tape:** Runs diagonally from the base of the cervical spine to a point on the upper third of the scapula (2). Your taping partner can pinpoint the base of the cervical spine by having you bend your head forward. The correct spot for attaching the tape will protrude when the head is bent.
- **Second strip of tape:** Runs horizontally from the upper end of the thoracic spine across the scapula (2).

Tip: Do a preliminary stretching of the muscles and joints so you can measure the length of the tape strips exactly.

Preliminary Stretching and Attachment of the Tape

Preliminary Stretching

- Move the arm on the side that is being taped across the front of your body to the other side and grip your opposite shoulder. Tilt your head slightly away from the side that is being taped, while simultaneously turning your chin a little bit toward the side that is being taped. Make sure that your back muscles are stretched (1).

Attaching the Tape

- The first strip of tape is attached at the protrusion of the bone at the base of the cervical spine that is visible and can be felt when the head is bent forward. The strip of tape runs in a slightly diagonal direction to the middle of the top third of the scapula (2).
- The second strip is put on slightly lower than the first strip, starting at the top of the thoracic spine. It is attached a little further across the scapula than the first strip of tape, which it should overlap a little (2).

Please Note

- If you stretch the rhomboid muscle tape slightly before attaching it, the stretched tape will make it easier to for the muscle to stretch.

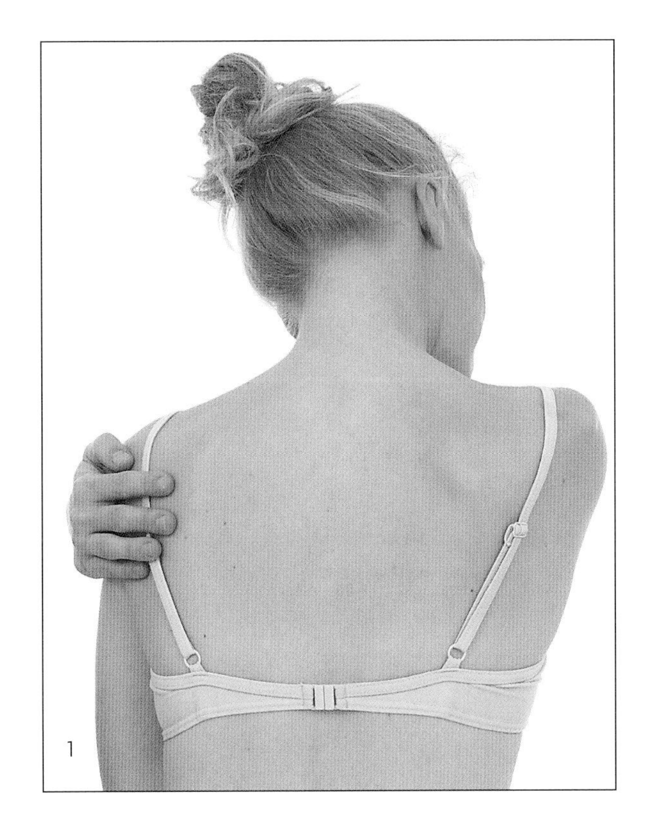

1

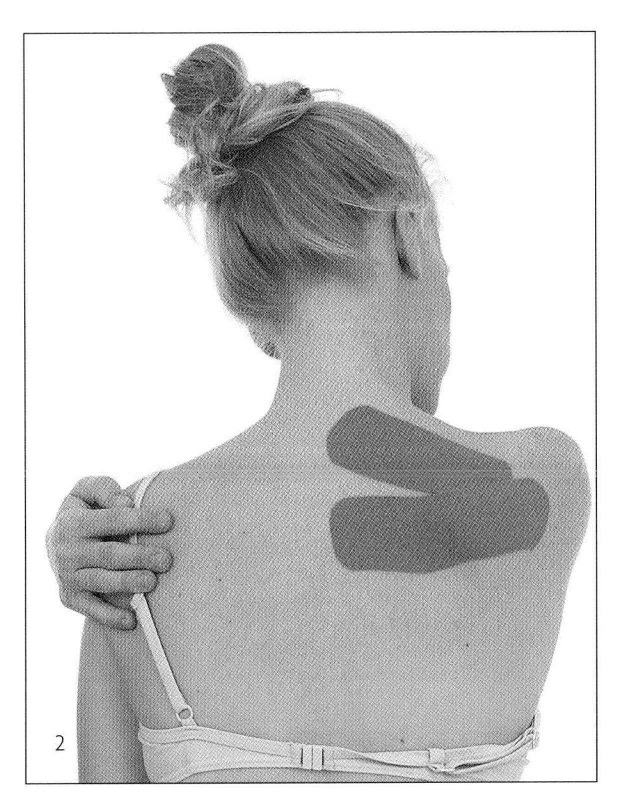

2

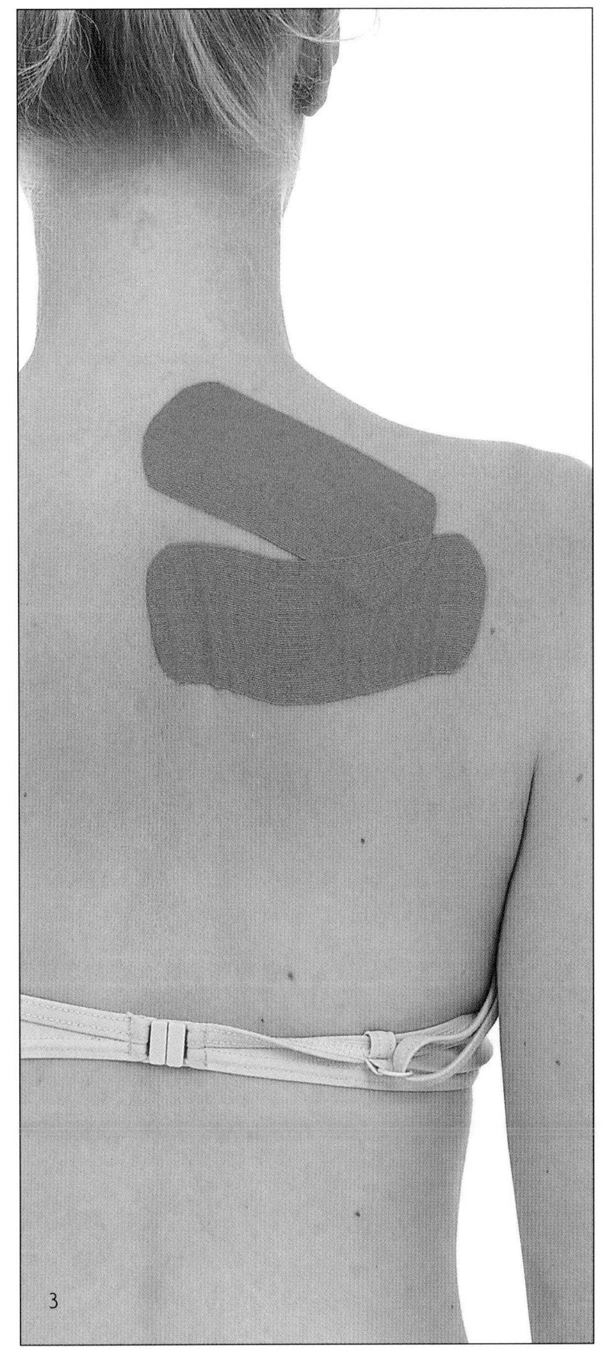

3

12. Cervical Spine Tape

Ailments

- Pain in the area of the cervical spine
- Headaches
- Dizziness
- Ringing in the ear (tinnitus)
- Pain in the area of the elbow
- Tennis elbow
- Golfer's elbow
- Pain in the area of the wrist
- Carpal tunnel syndrome (numbness in the area of the hand)

Number and Length of Tapes

Number of Tapes: 2

Measuring the Tape

- **First strip of tape:** Runs from the upper thoracic spine to the hairline (3).

Important: Three quarters of the length of the tape should be cut down the middle with a pair of scissors. Both ends should be rounded off (2).

- **Second strip of tape:** Runs from the middle of the right shoulder, across the back just below the neck, to the middle of the left shoulder (5).

Important: Fold the second strip of tape at the halfway point of its length and crease it well so that you can clearly see its middle point.

Tip: Do a preliminary stretching of the muscles and joints so you can measure the length of the tape strips exactly.

Preliminary Stretching and Attachment of the Tape

Preliminary Stretching

- Bend your head forward with your chin reaching as far as possible toward the breastbone, which will make the vertebral process at the base of the cervical spine visible (1).

Attaching the Tape

- Attach the first strip of tape at the upper part of the thoracic spine, beginning with the uncut end (2). Attach the left portion of the cut strip of tape on the left side of the spine up to the hairline, slightly left of center (3).

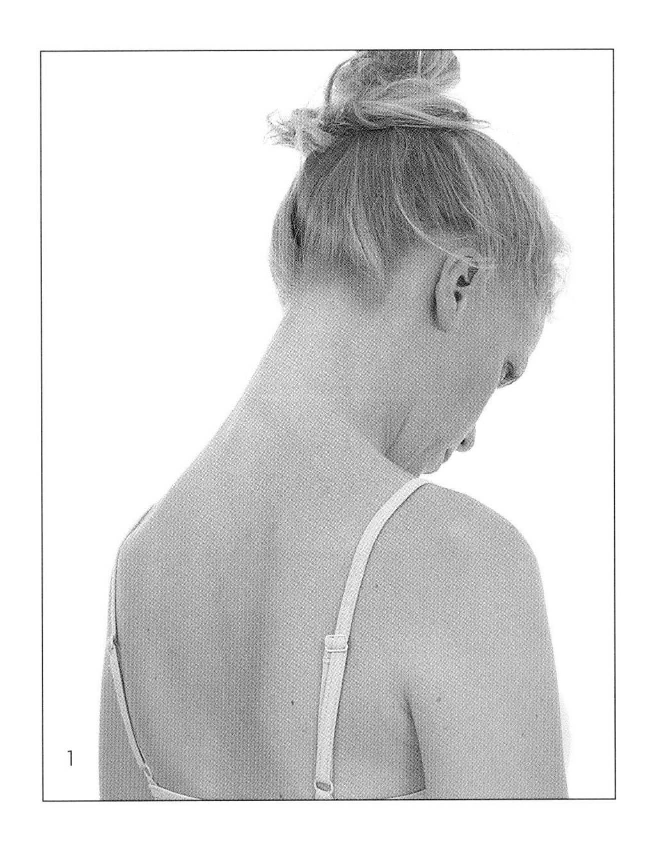
1

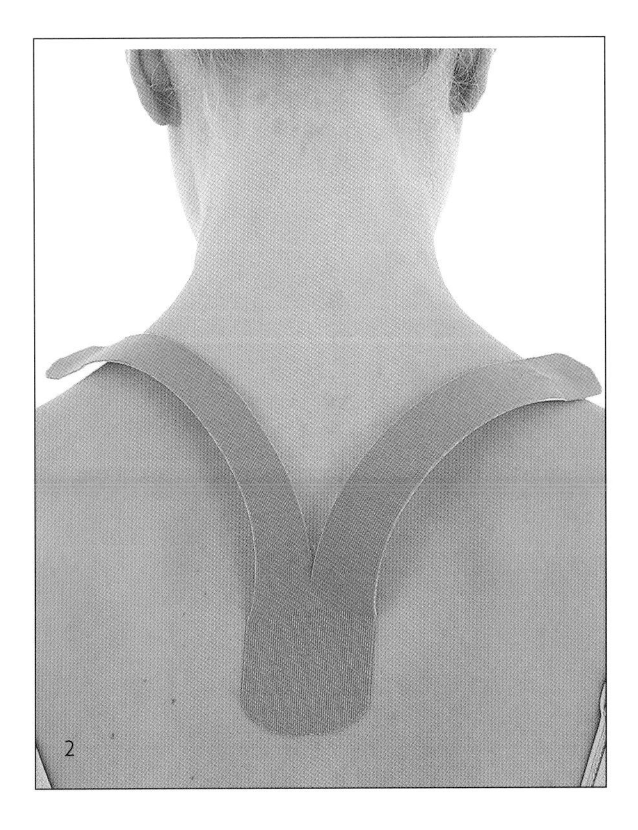
2

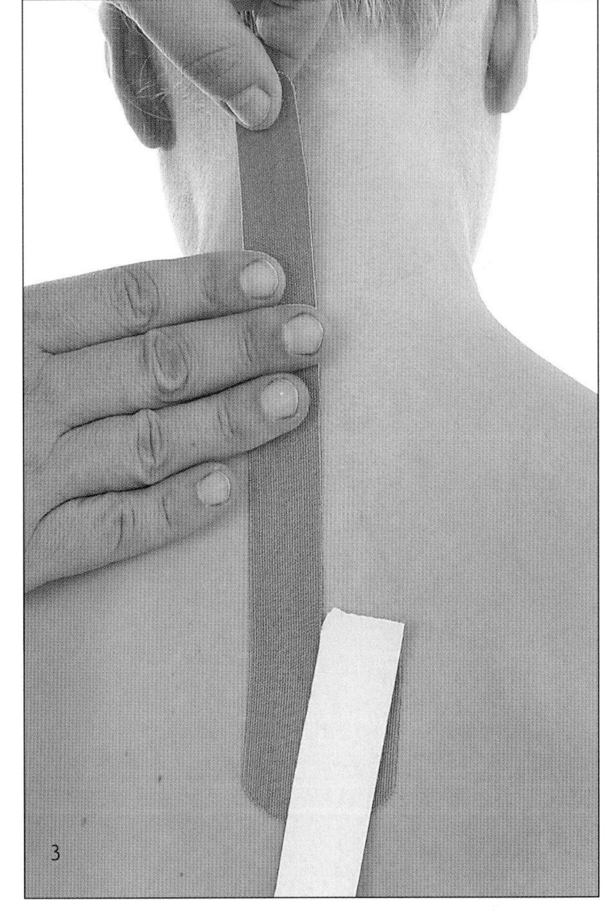
3

- Attach the right portion of the cut tape on the right side of the spine up to the hairline, slightly right of center (4).
- Attach the second strip of tape across the first strip at the transition from the cervical spine to the thoracic spine. The vertebral process of the cervical spine can be seen or felt easily as described in the preliminary stretching instructions. Use the middle fold on the second strip of tape to center it on the vertebral process. Attach the tape in a curve running right and left to the middle of each shoulder (5).

Please Note

- The transition points between the different regions of the spine are prone to disorders, so it is important that the second strip of tape completely cover the area of transition from the cervical spine to the thoracic spine.
- The cervical spine tape can also be used with the two strips of cervical spine lymph tape (see pages 72 and 73).

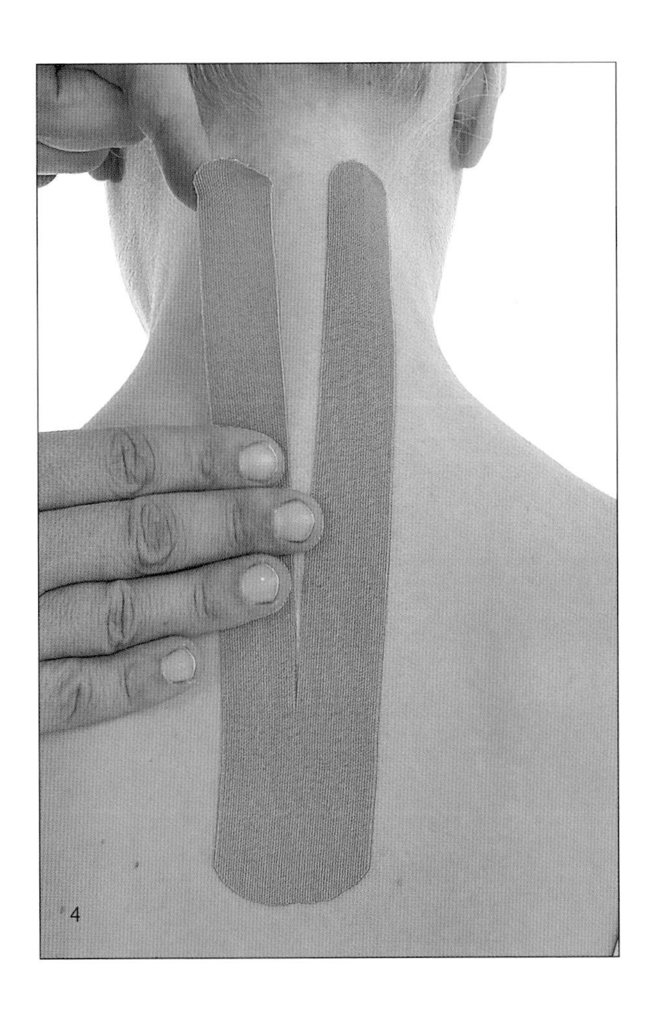

4

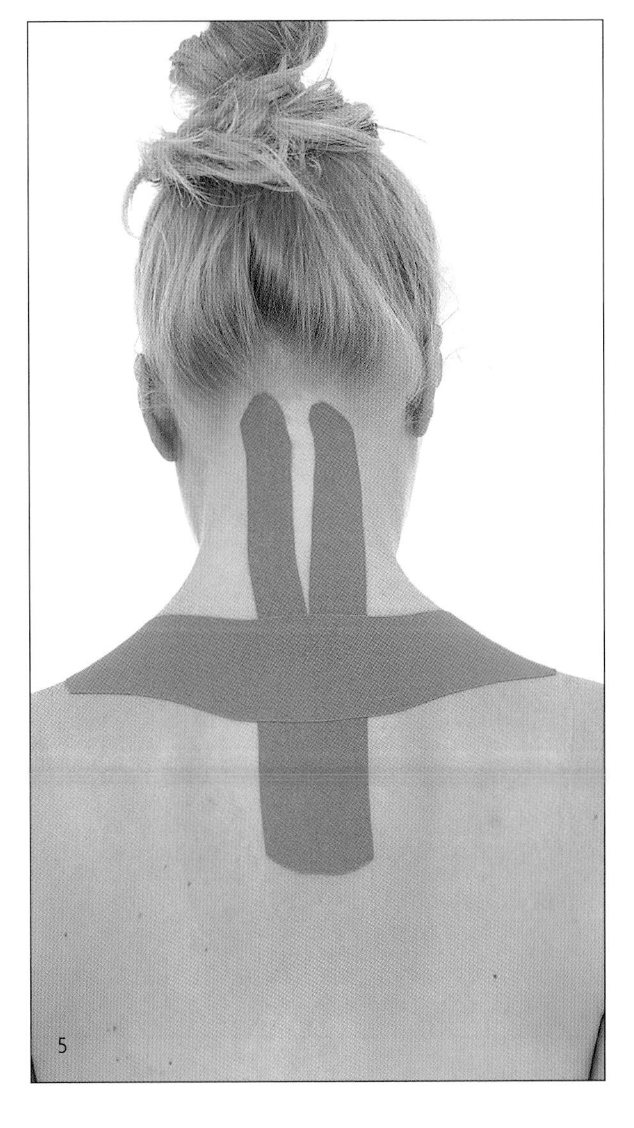

5

13. Cervical Spine Lymph Tape

Ailments

- Pain in the area of the cervical spine
- Headaches
- Sinusitis
- Hay fever
- Dizziness
- Ringing in the ears (tinnitus)

Number and Length of Tapes

Number of Tapes: 4

Measuring the Tape

- **First strip of tape:** Runs from the upper thoracic spine straight up to the hairline (see photo 3, page 69).

Important: Three quarters of the length of the tape should be cut down the middle with a pair of scissors and divided (see photo 2, page 69). Both ends of the split tape should be rounded off.

- **Second strip of tape:** Runs from the middle of the right shoulder, across the back just below the neck, to the middle of the left shoulder (1).

Important: Fold the second strip of tape at the halfway point of its length and crease it well so that you can clearly see its middle point.

- **Third strip of tape:** Runs from the middle of the left scapula up to the hairline, slightly left of center (2).
- **Fourth strip of tape:** Runs from the middle of the right scapula up to the hairline, slightly right of center (2).

Tip: Do a preliminary stretching of the muscles and joints so you can measure the length of the tape strips exactly.

Preliminary Stretching and Attachment of the Tape

Preliminary Stretching

- Tilt your head and chin as far as possible toward the breastbone (see photo 1, page 69).

Attaching the Tape

- Attach the first strip of tape at the upper part of the thoracic spine, beginning with the uncut end (see photo 2, page 69). Attach the left portion of the cut strip of tape on the left side of the spine up to the hairline, slightly left of center (see photo 3, page 69). Attach the right portion of the cut tape on the right side of the spine up to the hairline, slightly right of center (see photo 4, page 71).
- Attach the second strip of tape across the first strip at the transition from the cervical spine to the thoracic spine. The vertebral process of the cervical spine can be seen or felt easily as described in the preliminary stretching instructions for the cervical spine tape (page 68). Use the middle fold on the second strip of tape to center it on the vertebral process. Attach the tape in a curve running right and left to the middle of each shoulder (1).
- Attach the third strip of tape from the middle of the left scapula up to the hairline, slightly left of center (2).
- Attach the fourth strip tape from the middle of the right scapula up to the hairline, slightly right of center (2).

Please Note

- The cervical spine lymph tape is based on the cervical spine tape and complements that tape, when the two are used together, in the treatment of sinusitis and ailments like hay fever.

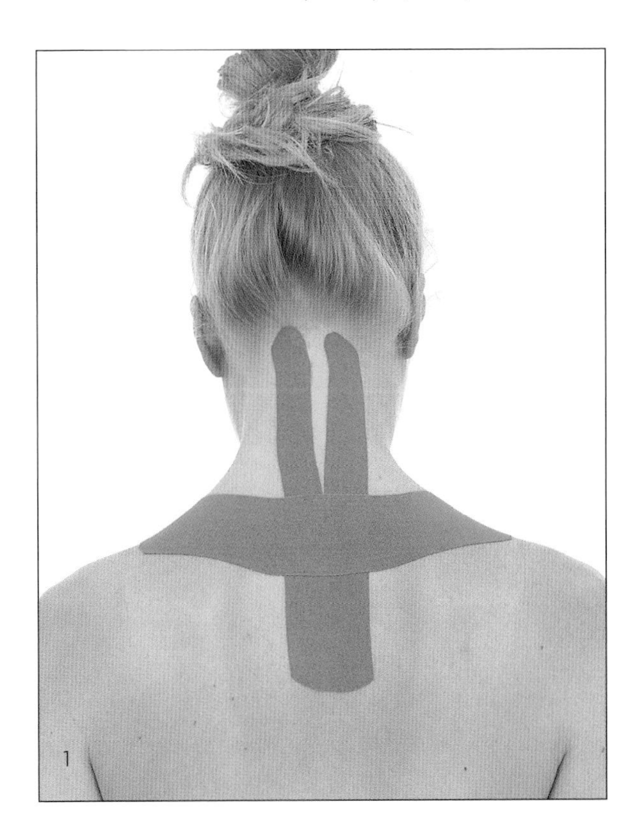
1

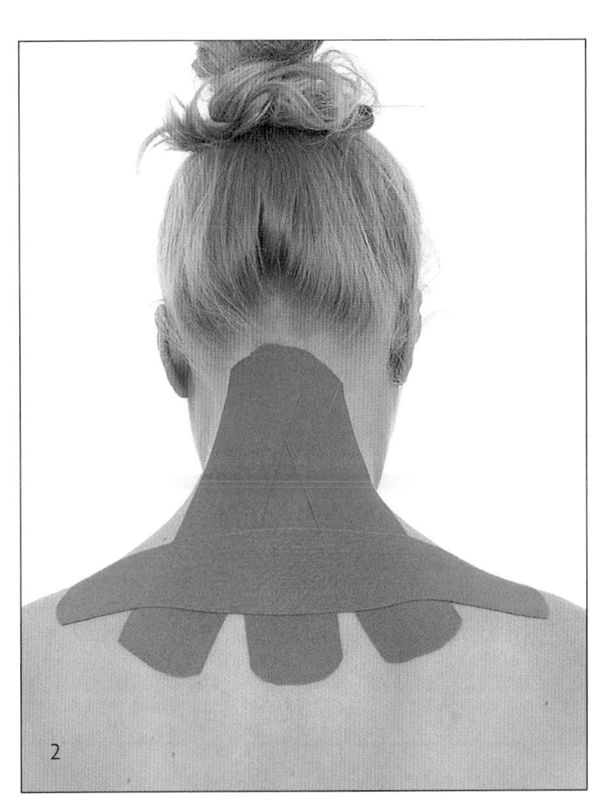
2

14. Thoracic Spine Tape

Ailments

- Pain in the area of the thoracic spine
- Pain in the chest
- Pain in the ribcage

Number and Length of Tapes

Number of Tapes: 2

Measuring the Tape

- Both strips of tape run from the transition point between the lumbar spine and the thoracic spine up to the base of the cervical spine (3).

Tip: Do a preliminary stretching of the muscles and joints so you can measure the length of the tape strips exactly!

Preliminary Stretching and Attachment of the Tape

Preliminary Stretching

- Sit on a stool or a chair. Tilt your head toward your breastbone as far as possible and curve your whole back forward (1).

Attaching the Tape

- Starting at the transition point between the lumbar spine and the thoracic spine, attach the first strip of tape along the left side of the spine. Run it straight up, nearly the whole length of the back, to the level of the vertebral process at the base of the cervical spine (2).
- Attach the second strip in the same way as the first, but on the right side of the spine (2).

Please Note

- It is important that you attach two whole strips of tape parallel to each other, rather than using half of a strip on each side. Cutting tapes down the middle is acceptable for some taping protocols but not in this case.

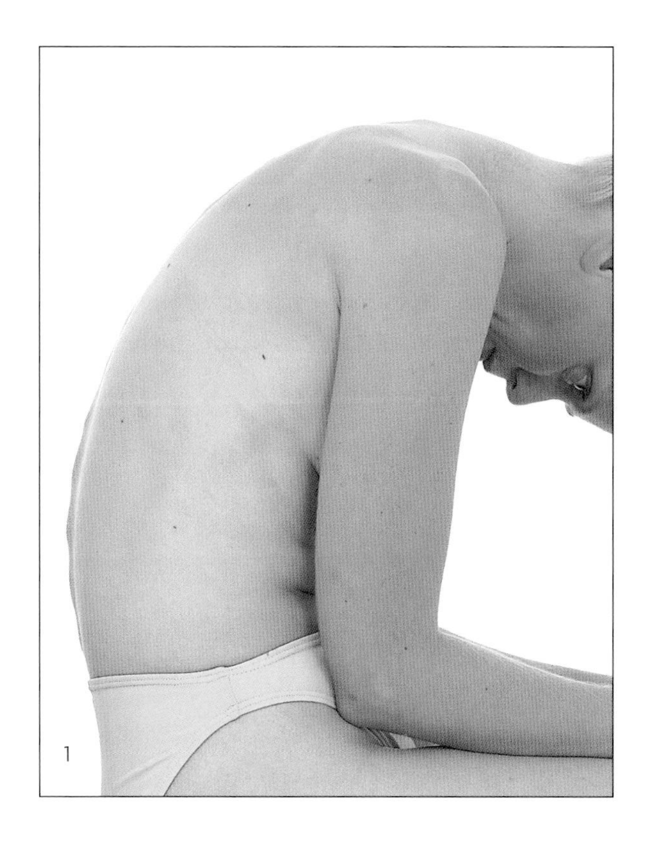
1

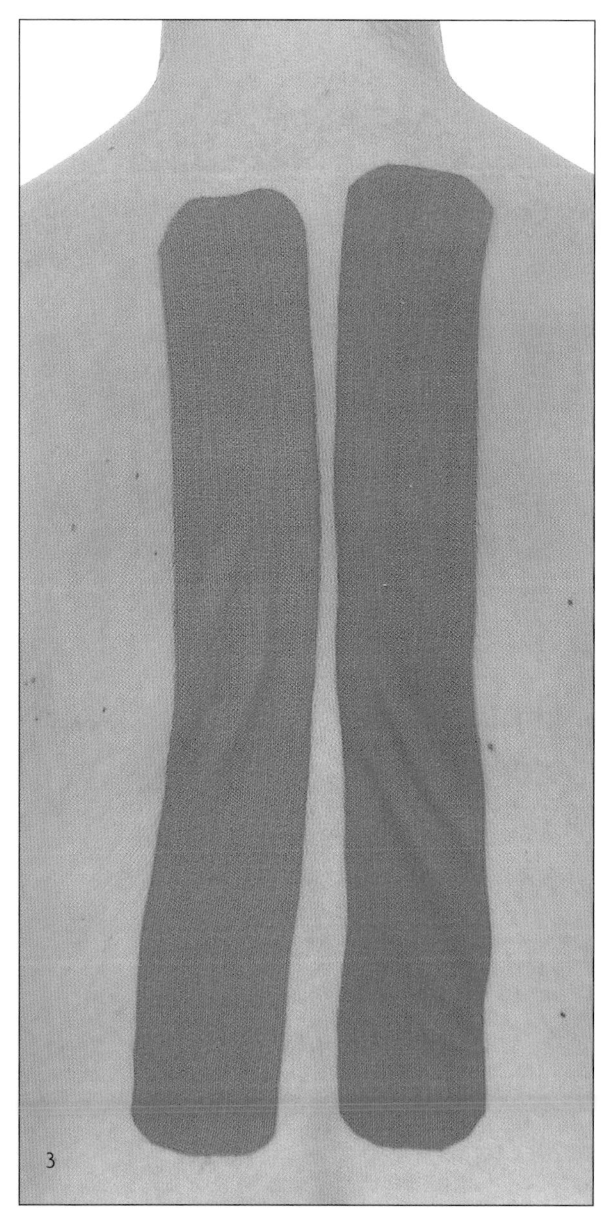
3

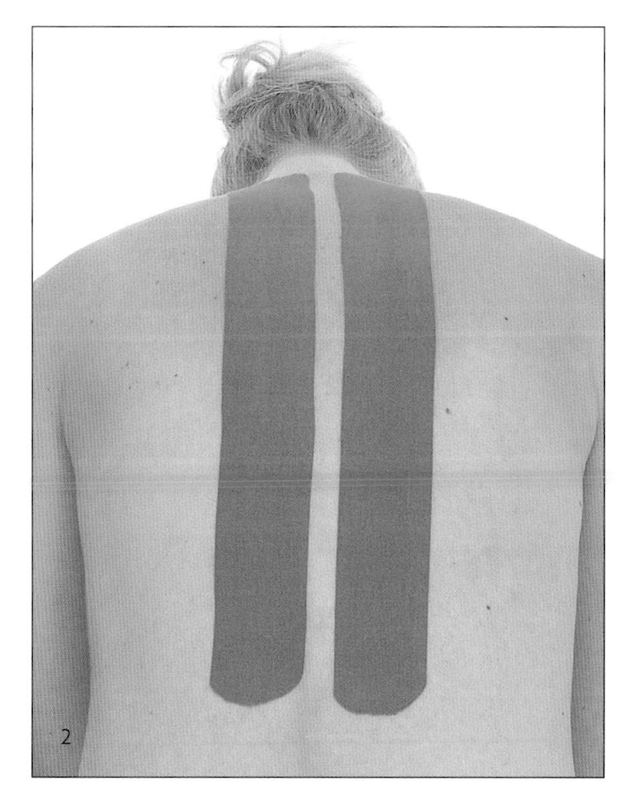
2

15. Lumbar Spine Tape

Ailments

- Pain in the area of the lumbar spine
- Pain in the area of the tailbone
- Pain in the hips
- Postoperative pain after surgery on a spinal disc
- Pain in the leg
- Restless legs syndrome
- Pain in the foot
- Menstrual pain
- Stomachache
- Discomfort in the area of the belly during pregnancy
- Digestive disorders
- Diarrhea
- Irritated bladder
- Incontinence

Number and Length of Tapes

Number of Tapes: 3

Measuring the Tape

- **First and second strips of tape:** Run on either side of the spine from the lower lumbar portion of the spine straight up to the base of the thoracic spine (2).
- **Third strip of tape:** Runs horizontally across the center of the back at the level of the upper lumbar spine (3).

Tip: Do a preliminary stretching of the muscles and joints so you can measure the length of the tape strips exactly.

Preliminary Stretching and Attachment of the Tape

Preliminary Stretching

- Sit on a stool or a chair. Tilt your head down toward your breastbone and curve your whole back forward (1).

Attaching the Tape

- Attach the first strip of tape on the right side of the lower lumbar spine and run it straight up to the base of the thoracic spine (2).
- Attach the second strip in the same way, beginning on the left side of the lower lumbar spine (2).
- Attach the third strip horizontally across the first two strips of tape at the level of the upper lumbar spine (3).

Please Note

- It is important that you attach two *whole* strips of tape parallel to each other, rather than using half of a strip on each side. Split tapes are acceptable for some taping protocols, but not in this case.
- The lumbar spine tape is more effective if the tape is attached all the way to the lower part of the thoracic spine.
- This tape can also be used with three more tape strips, as shown in the next section on the lumbar spine star tape (pages 78–81).

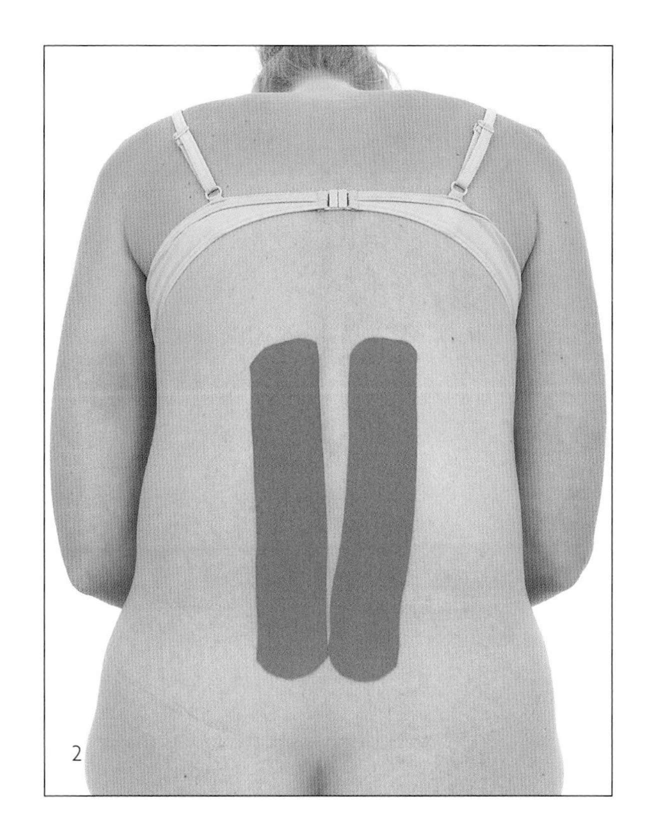

2

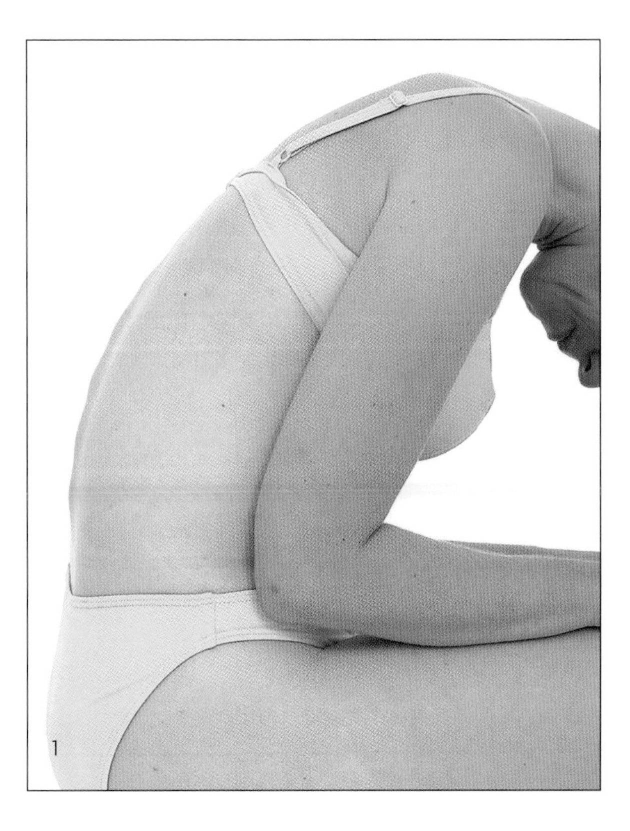

1

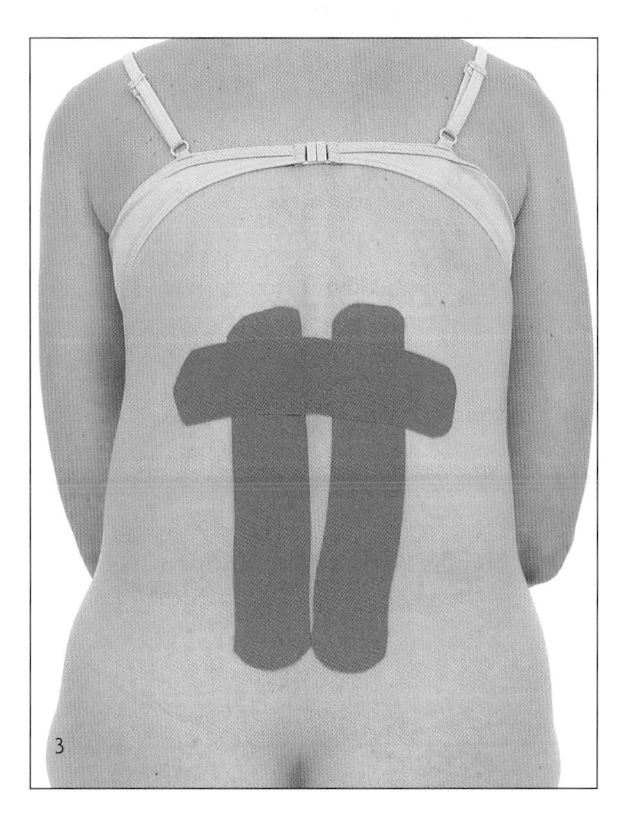

3

16. Lumbar Spine Star Tape

Ailments

- Pain in the area of the lumbar spine
- Menstrual pain
- Postoperative pain after surgery on a spinal disc

Number and Length of Tapes

Number of Tapes: 6

Measuring the Tape

- **First and second strips of tape:** Run on either side of the spine from the lower lumbar portion of the spine straight up to the base of the thoracic spine (2).
- **Third strip of tape:** Runs horizontally across the center of the back at the level of the upper lumbar spine (3).
- **Fourth, fifth, and sixth strips of tape:** Attach the last three strips of tape in a star formation in the area of the lower lumbar spine, with one strip running horizontally across and the other two running in both diagonal directions (4, 5).

Important: The last three tape strips should be gently stretched before you attach them.

Tip: Do a preliminary stretching of the muscles and joints so you can measure the length of the tape strips exactly.

Preliminary Stretching and Attachment of the Tape

Preliminary Stretching

- Sit on a stool or a chair. Tilt your head down toward your breastbone and curve your whole back forward (1).

Attaching the Tape

- Attach the first strip of tape on the right side of the lower lumbar spine and run it straight up to the base of the thoracic spine (2).
- Attach the second strip in the same way, beginning on the left side of the lower lumbar spine (2).
- Attach the third strip horizontally across the first two strips of tape at the level of the upper lumbar spine (3).

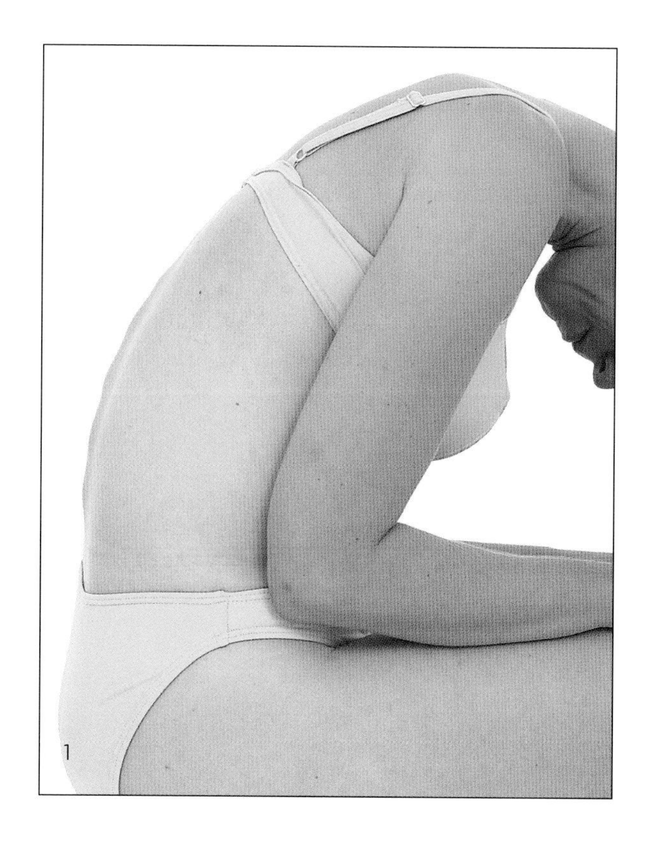
1

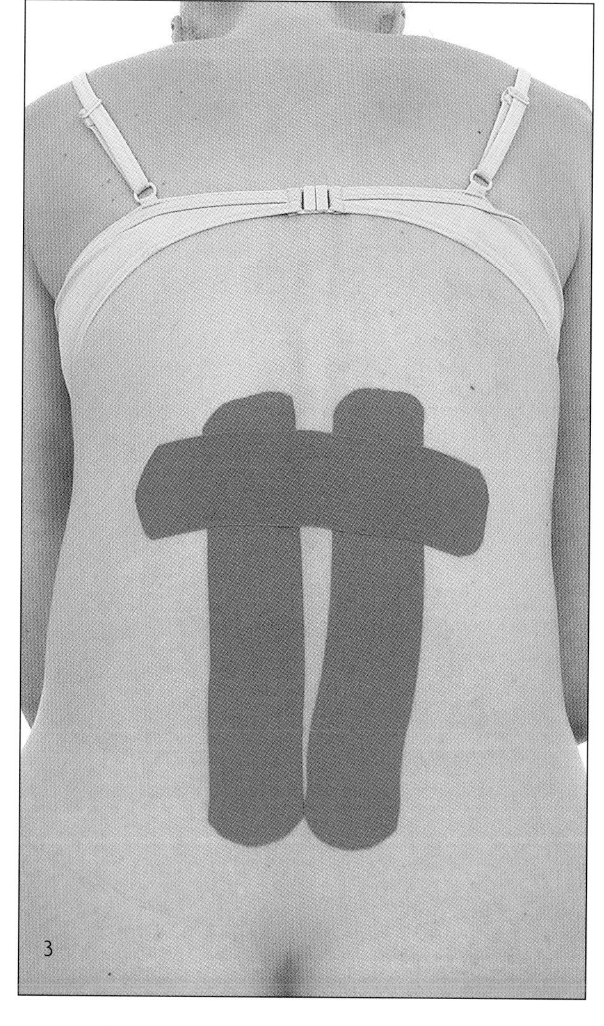
3

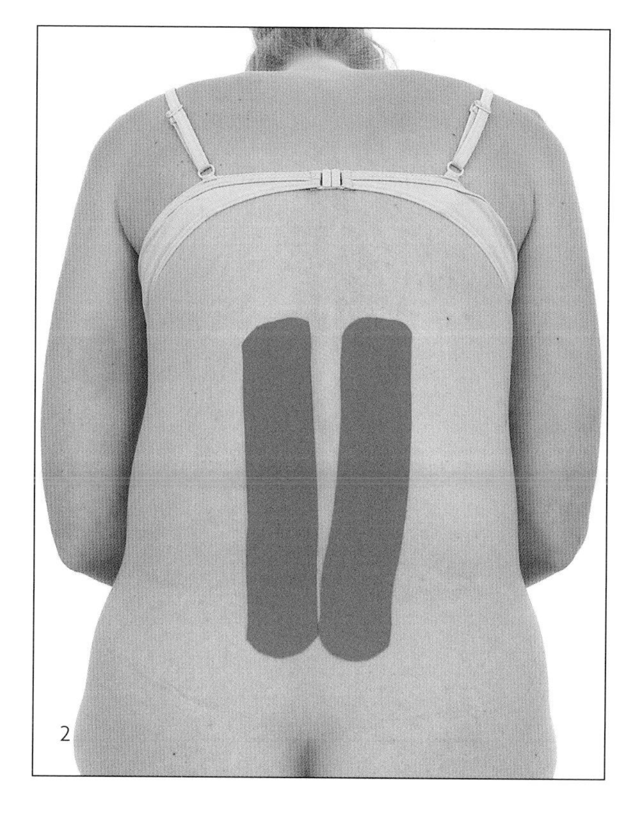
2

- Stretch the fourth strip and attach it horizontally across the lower lumbar spine and over the first two tapes (4).
- Stretch the fifth and sixth strips as well and attached in an "X" over the fourth strip (5).

Please Note

- Although the fourth, fifth, and sixth strips of tape should be stretched slightly, you should not stretch the first three strips—or do so only very, very slightly.
- The tape is more efficient if the first two strips of tape are run up to the area of the lower thoracic spine.
- The two vertical strips are attached parallel to each other—so please use two tapes. Do not use one strip cut into two halves. Split tape is acceptable for some acutaping protocols, but not for this one.

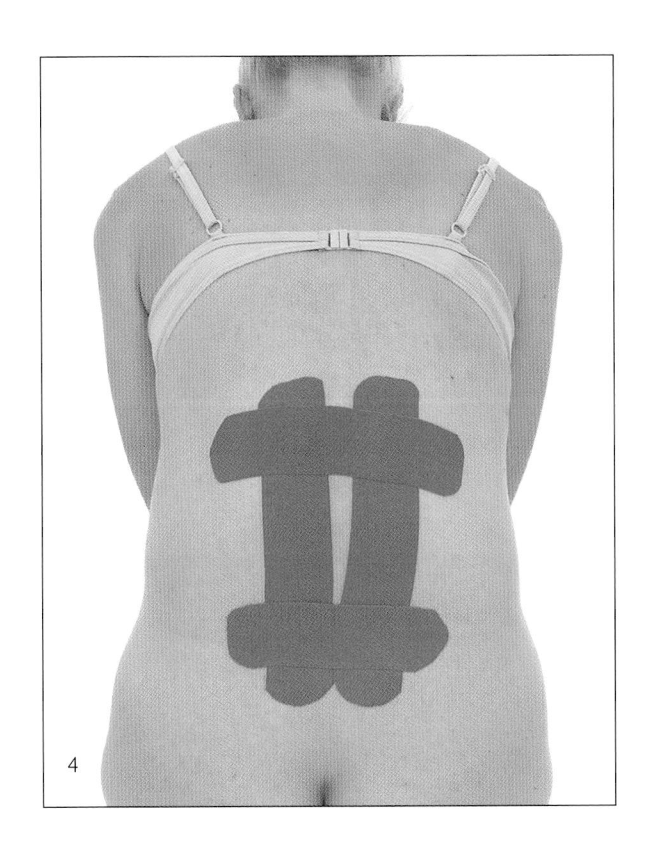

4

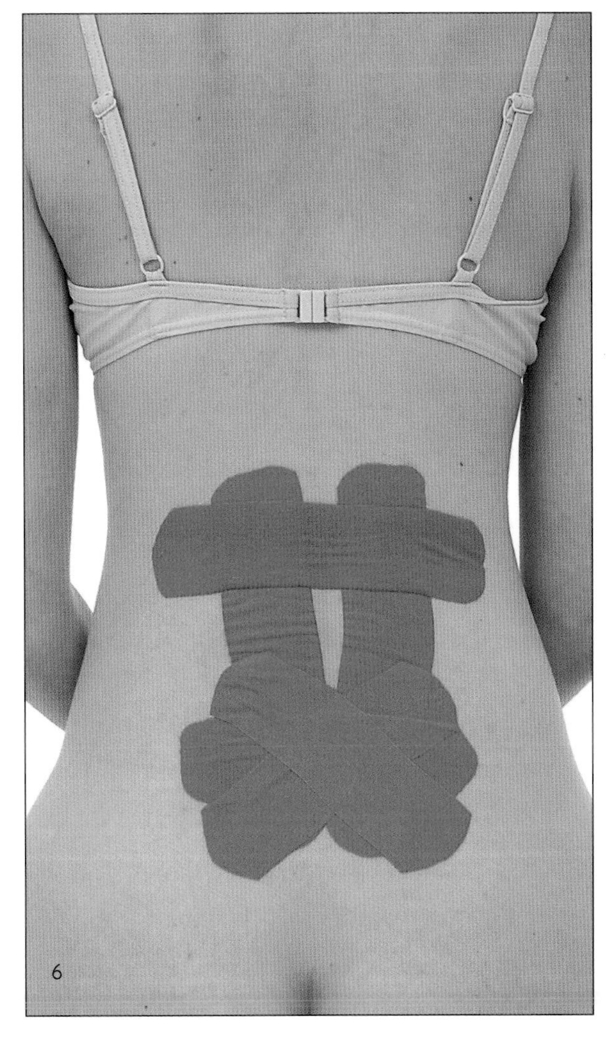

6

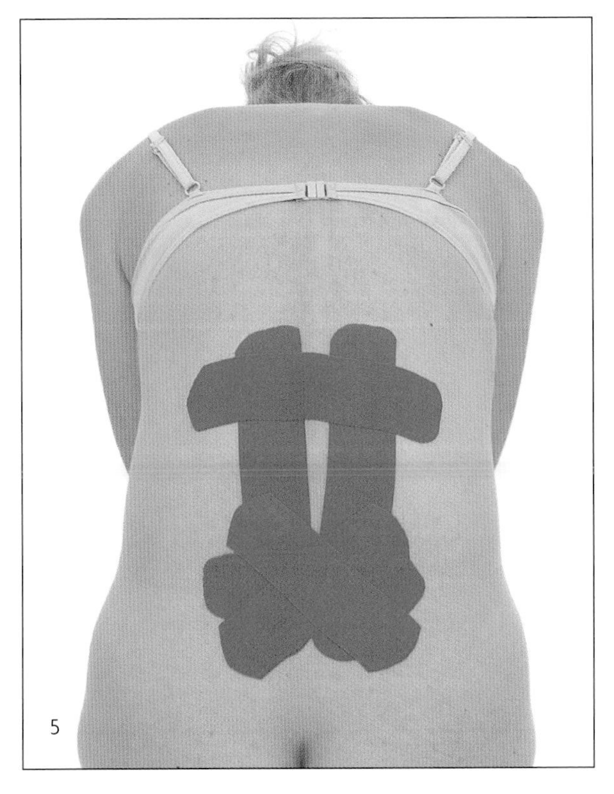

5

17. Sacroiliac Joint Tape

Ailments

- Pain in the area of the lumbar spine
- Pain in the tailbone (coccyx)
- Pain in the hips
- Menstrual pain
- Headaches
- Irritated bladder
- Dizziness
- Ringing of the ears (tinnitus)

Number and Length of Tapes

Number of Tapes: 4

Measuring the Tape

- **First and second strips of tape:** Cover two-thirds of the length of the lumbar spine (1, 2).
- **Third and fourth strips of tape:** Run from the fold between the buttocks outward to the hip (4, 5).

Tip: Do a preliminary stretching of the muscles and joints so you can measure the length of the tape strips exactly.

Preliminary Stretching and Attachment of the Tape

First Strip of Tape

- **Preliminary stretching:** Sit on a stool or a chair, tilt your head down, and curve your whole back forward (1).
- **Attaching the tape:** Attach the tape vertically next to the lumbar spine, starting a little above the fold between the buttocks and running up to the upper third of the lumbar spine (1).

Second Strip of Tape

- **Preliminary stretching:** Sit up straight; bend the upper part of your body away from the side that is being taped; and put your hand from the side that is being taped on the top of your head (2).
- **Attaching the tape:** Stretch the second strip of tape a little before attaching it. Put it next to the first tape, a little farther away from the spine and a little higher up the back, in the direction of the thoracic spine (2). The two strips of tape should overlap.

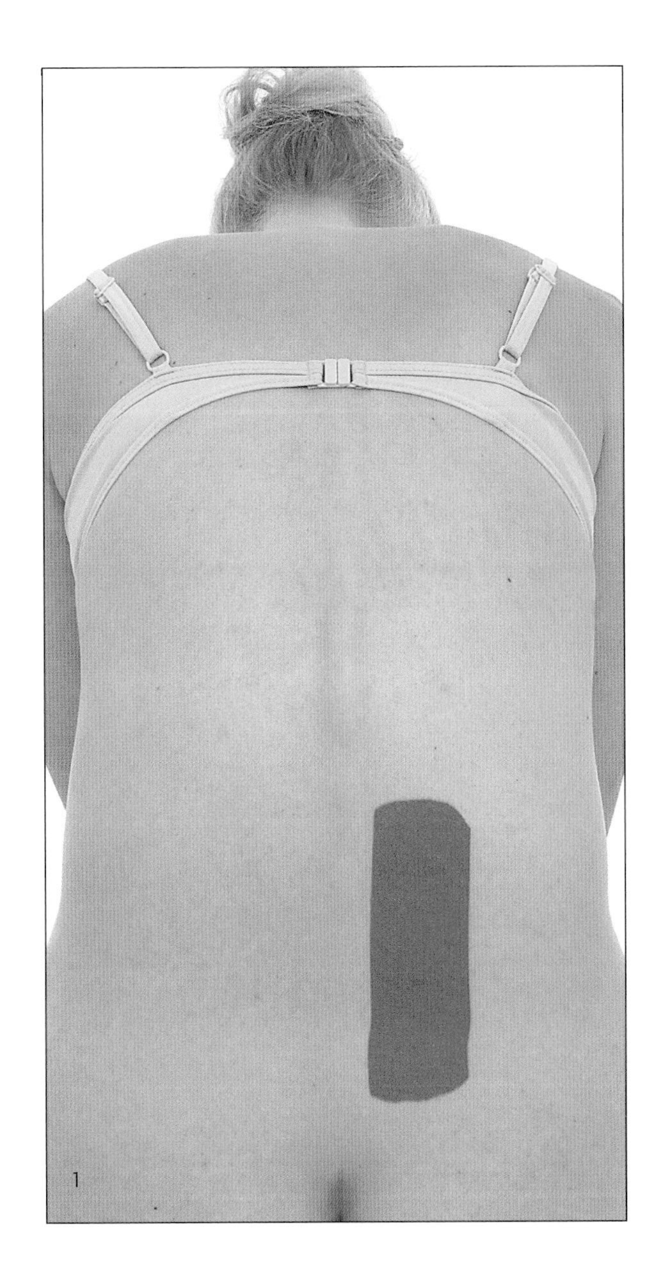
1

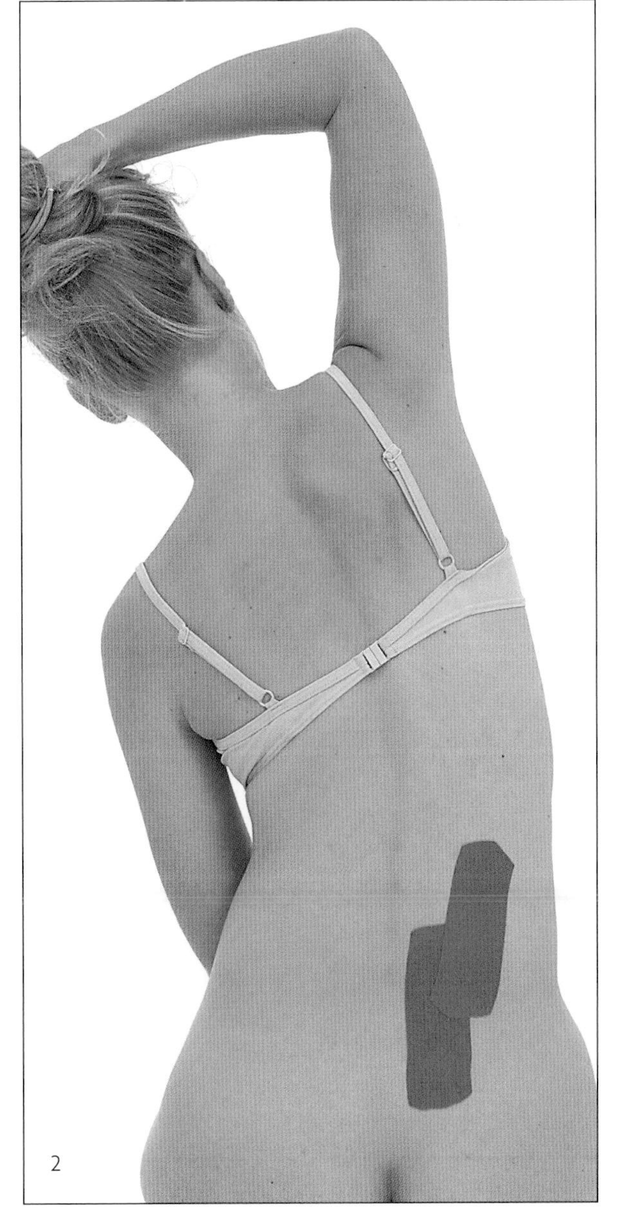
2

Third and Fourth Strips of Tape

- **Preliminary stretching:** Recline on the side that is not being taped, stretch the lower leg out, and bend the upper leg at the hip joint until the thigh is even with the hip (3).
- **Attaching the tape:** Attach the third strip of tape a little above the fold between the buttocks. Run it along the top of the buttock and over the hip (3).
- Attach the fourth strip from the tip of the fold between the buttocks. Run it across the curve of the buttock and over the hip (4). The third and fourth strips should overlap at the hip.

Please Note

- Disturbances of the sacroiliac joint play an important role in many ailments. Thus, when chronic conditions are treated, it is recommended that the sacroiliac joint be taped along with any other acutaping treatment.

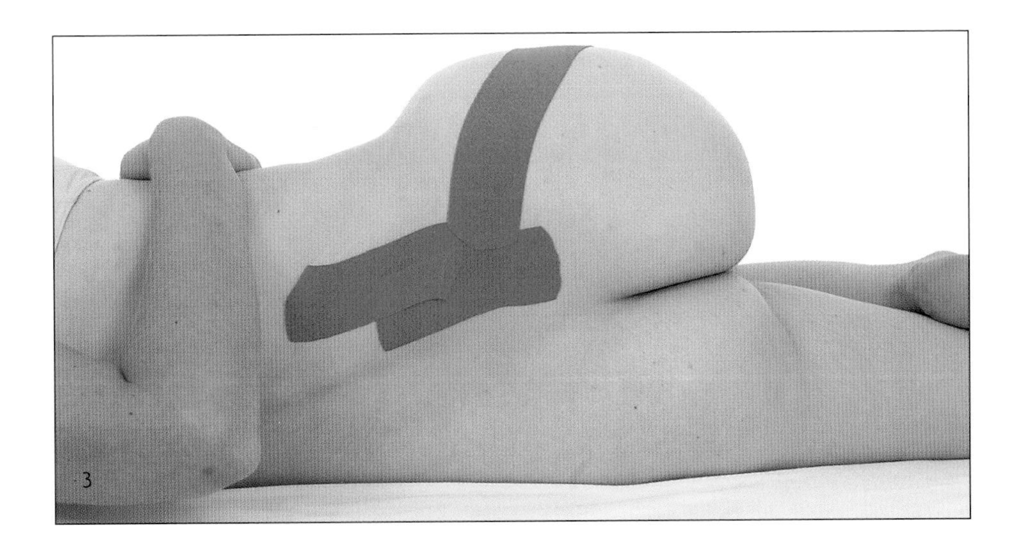
3

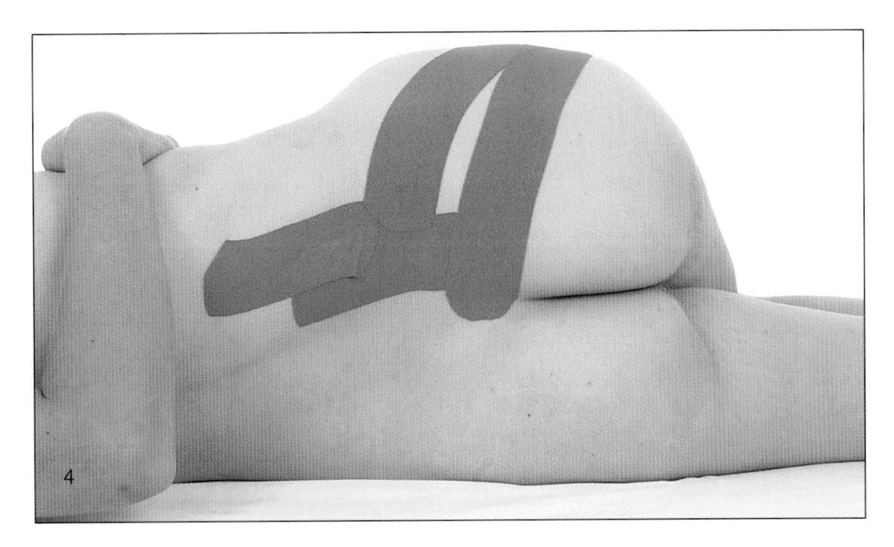
4

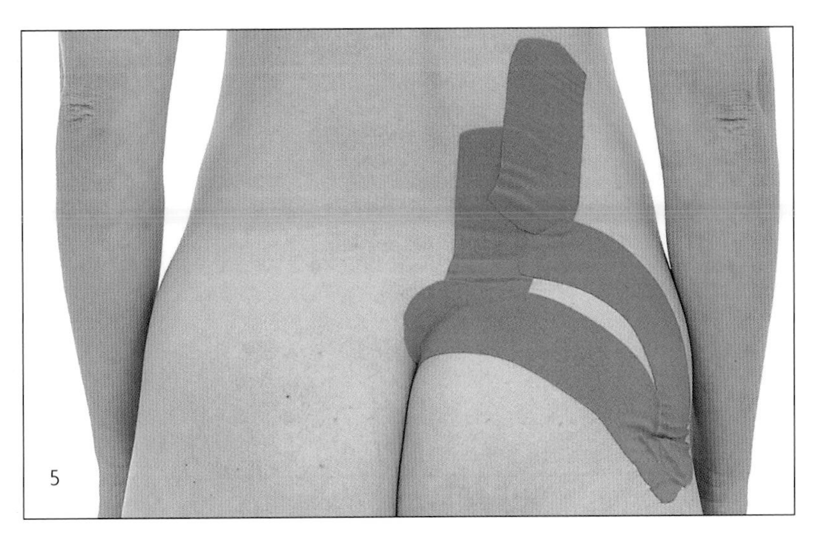
5

18. Abdominal Muscle Tape (Rectus Abdominus)

Ailments

- Stomachache
- Ailments during pregnancies in the area of the belly
- Menstrual pain
- Indigestion
- Diarrhea
- Constipation
- Irritated bladder
- Incontinence

Number and Length of Tapes

Number of Tapes: 2

Measuring the Tape

- Both strips of tape run from the upper border of the pubic hair straight up to the lowest edge of the rib cage, which can be easily felt, ending near the point where the ribs meet the breastbone (2).

Tip: Do a preliminary stretching of the muscles and joints so you can measure the length of the tape strips exactly.

Preliminary Stretching and Attachment of the Tape

Preliminary Stretching

- Sit on a big armchair or a bed. Bend the upper part of your body back and, while supporting yourself with your arms on the bed or chair, thrust your pelvis toward the front (1).

Attaching the Tape

- Attach the first strip of tape to the left of the body's midline. Run it from the upper border of the pubic hair to the lower edge of the rib cage near the point where the rib meets the breastbone (2).
- The second strip of tape is attached to the right of the body's midline, parallel to the first strip (2).

Please Note

- The preliminary stretching needed for this taping might not be possible for everyone. The tape also can be attached while you are reclining. Put a pillow or other soft support underneath the thoracic spine to create a little preliminary stretching.

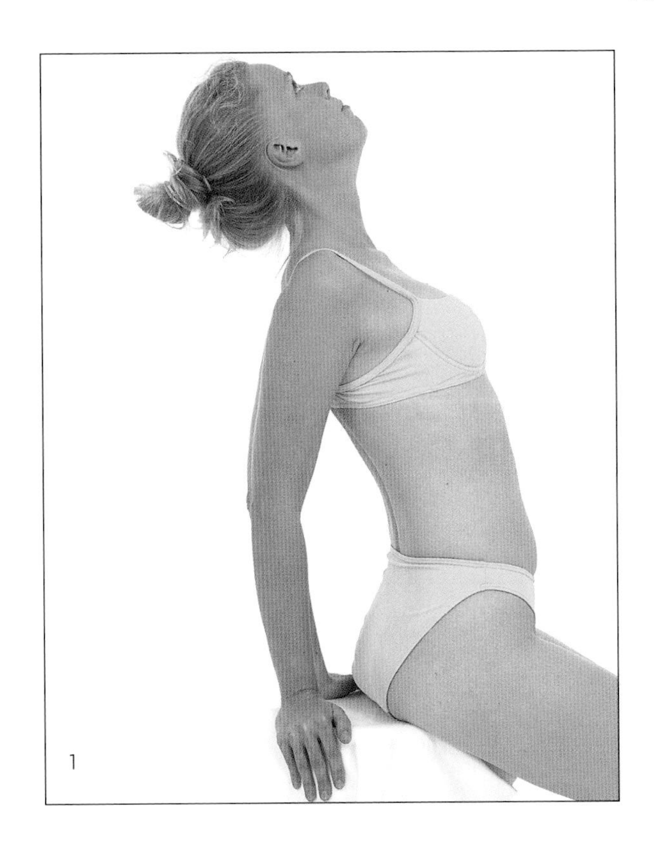
1

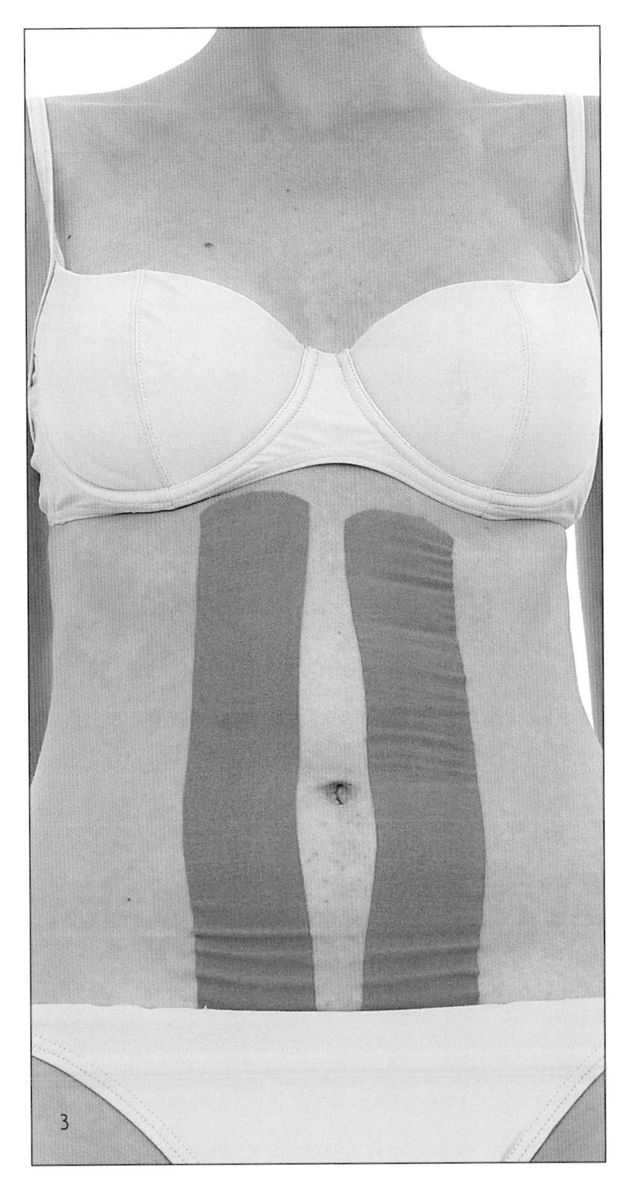
3

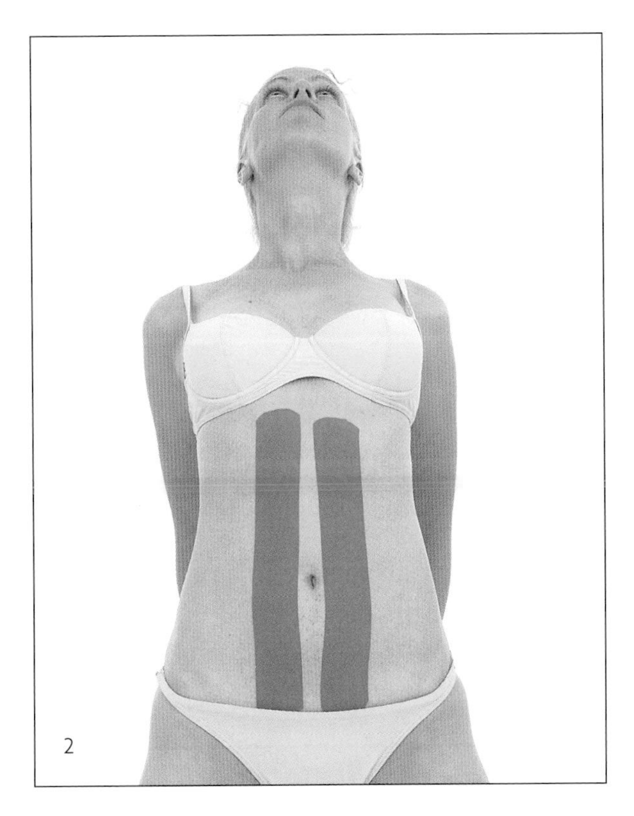
2

19. Abdominal Muscle Tape (Oblique Muscles)

Ailments

- Stomachache
- Ailment in the area of the belly during pregnancy
- Menstrual pain
- Digestive ailments
- Diarrhea
- Constipation
- Irritated bladder
- Incontinence

Number and Length of Tapes

Number of Tapes: 4

Measuring the Tape

- **First and third strips of tape:** Runs from beneath the ribs on the side of the body diagonally down to the groin, closer to the midline of the body. Repeat on opposite side (1).
- **Second and fourth strips of tape:** Runs from the groin diagonally up the abdomen, following the angle of the rib cage where it meets the breastbone, which can be easily felt beneath the breast. Repeat on the opposite side (2).

Tip: Do a preliminary stretching of the muscles and joints so you can measure the length of the tape strips exactly!

Preliminary Stretching and Attachment of the Tape

Preliminary Stretching of the Right Side

- Sitting on the edge of a bed, bend the upper part of your body back, and turn your right shoulder slightly more to the back (1).

Attaching the Tape on the Right Side

- Attach the first strip of tape on the right side of the body beneath the rib cage and run it down to the groin, ending to the right of the body's midline.
- Attach the second strip on the right side of the groin. Run it diagonally along the abdomen, ending near the bend of the rib cage where it turns to meets the breastbone (2).

Preliminary Stretching of the Left Side

- Turn the left shoulder toward the back.

Attaching the Tape on the Left Side

- Attach the first strip of tape on the left side of the body beneath the rib cage and run it down to the groin, ending to the left of the body's midline (1).
- Attach the second strip on the left side of the groin. Run it diagonally along the abdomen, ending near the bend of the rib cage where the rib meets the breastbone (2).

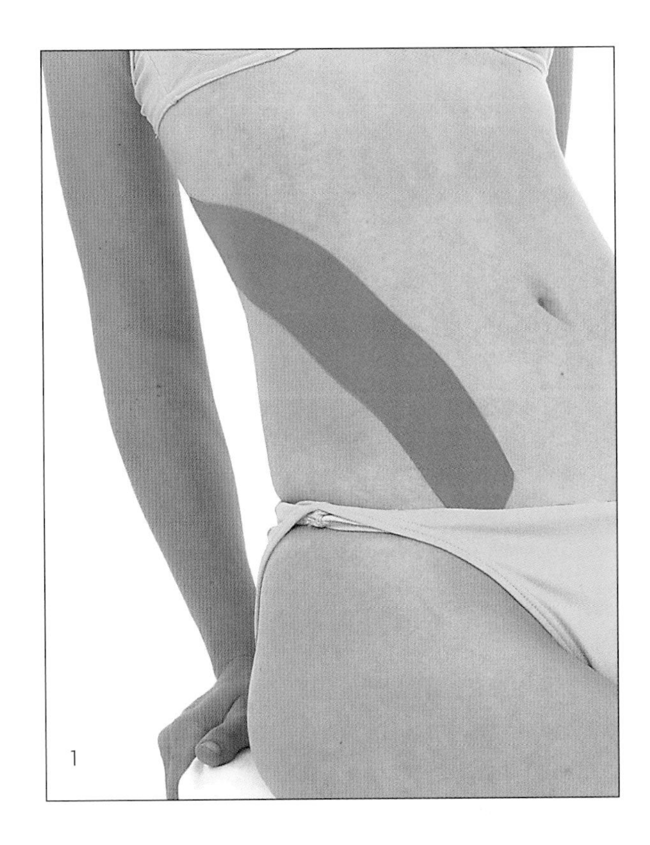
1

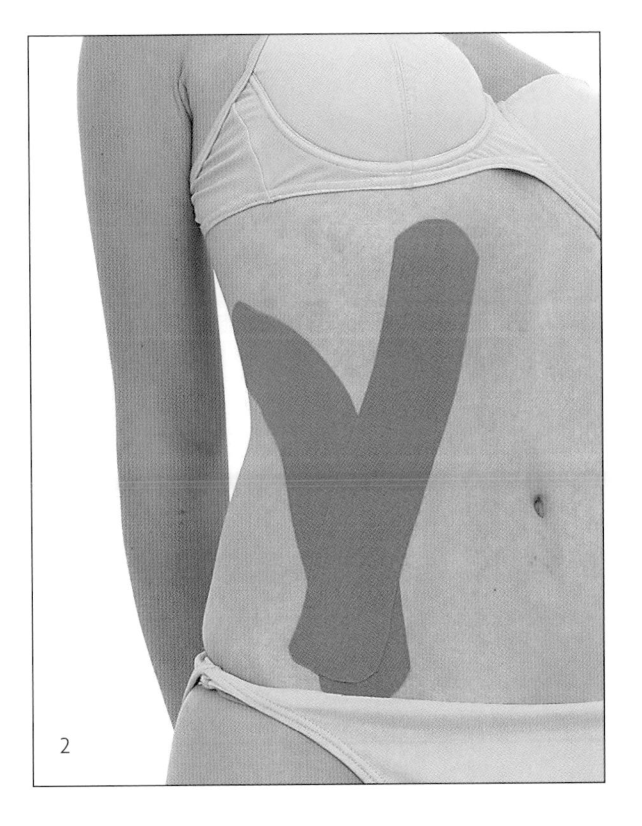
2

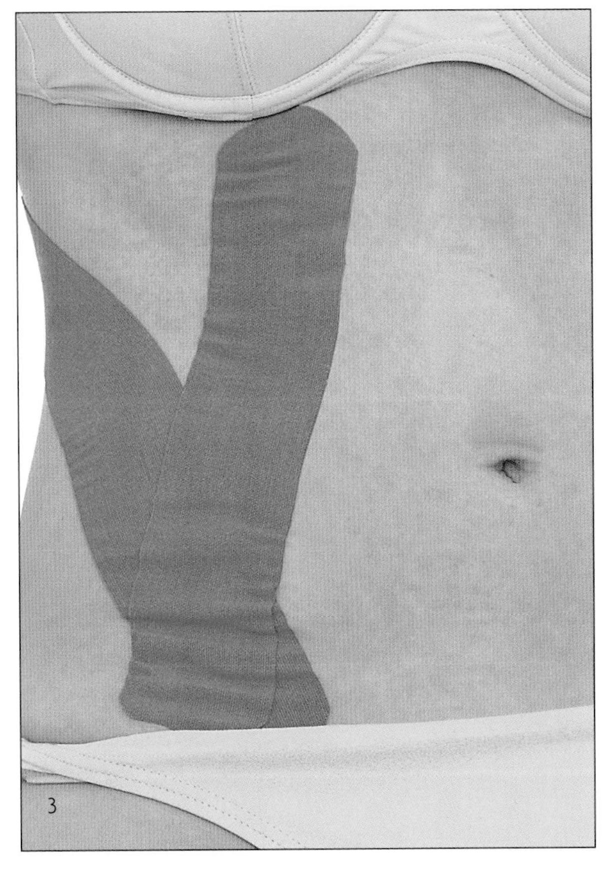
3

20. Pelvic Bone Muscle Tape

Ailments

- Pain in the tailbone
- Pain in the hips
- Pain in the legs
- Pain in the area of the thoracic spine and lumbar spine

Number and Length of Tapes

Number of Tapes: 1

Measuring the Tape

- The tape strip runs from the inner side of the thigh, a little below the pelvis, and crosses diagonally over the groin to end below the hipbone (2).

Tip: Do a preliminary stretching of the muscles and joints so you can measure the length of the tape strips exactly.

Important: Slightly stretch the strip of tape before attaching it.

Preliminary Stretching and Attachment of the Tape

Preliminary Stretching

- Recline on a table so that your leg on the side being taped hangs down next to the table with the knee bent. Bend the other leg up, hold it with both hands on the shin, and pull the leg toward your body (1).

Attaching the Tape

- Attach the prestretched strip of tape to the inner side of the thigh, a little below the pelvis, and run it diagonally across the groin to end below the hipbone (2).

Please Note

- To intensify the preliminary stretching, you can rotate the leg on the side being taped slightly more toward the inside of the hip joint.

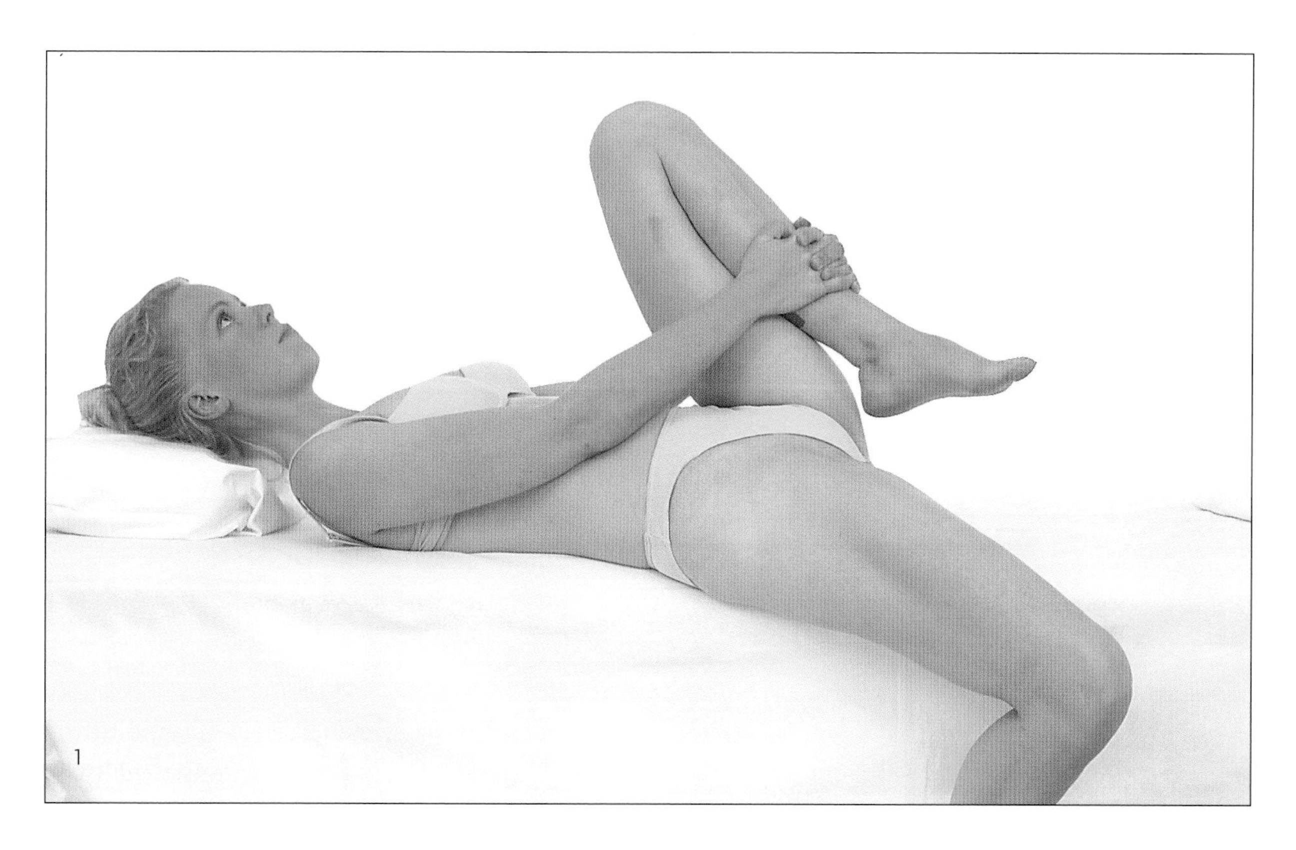
1

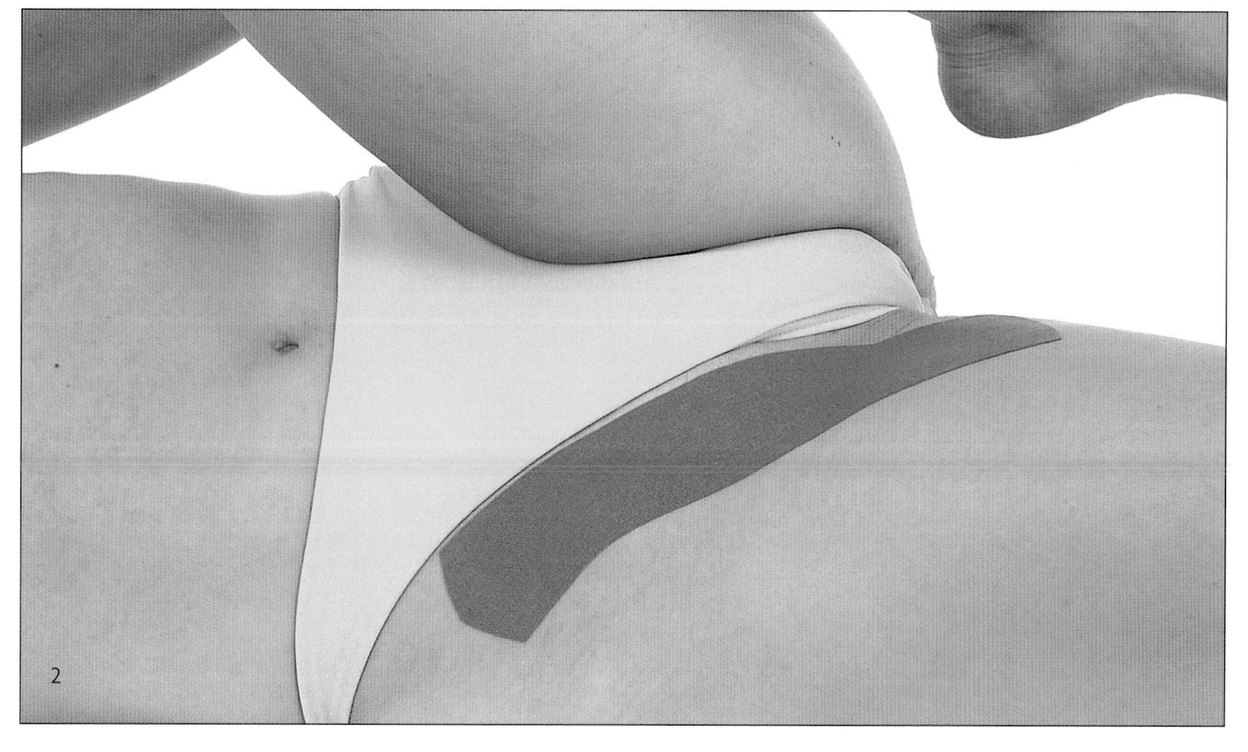
2

21. Hip and Loin Flexor (Iliopsoas) Muscle Tape

Ailments

- Pain in the hips
- Pain in the legs
- Pain in the thoracic and lumbar spine

Number and Length of Tapes

Number of Tapes: 1

Measuring the Tape

- The tape strip runs at an angle down the abdomen from a point halfway between the navel and the bend of the rib cage where the lowest rib approaches the breastbone (easily felt beneath the breast), passing over the groin to end on the inner side of the thigh (2).

Tip: Do a preliminary stretching of the muscles and joints so you can measure the length of the tape strips exactly.

Important: Slightly stretch the strip of tape before attaching!

Preliminary Stretching and Attachment of the Tape

Preliminary Stretching

- Recline on a table so that your leg on the side being taped hangs down next to the table with the knee bent. Bend the other leg up, hold it with both hands on the shin, and pull the leg toward your body (1).

Attaching the Tape

- Attach the prestretched strip of tape in the middle of the body at a point halfway between the navel and the bend of the rib cage where the lowest rib approaches the breastbone (easily felt underneath the breast). From this point the tape runs at an angle down the abdomen to the groin and the inner side of the thigh (2).

Please Note

- In medical terminology, this tape is also called iliopsoas tape.

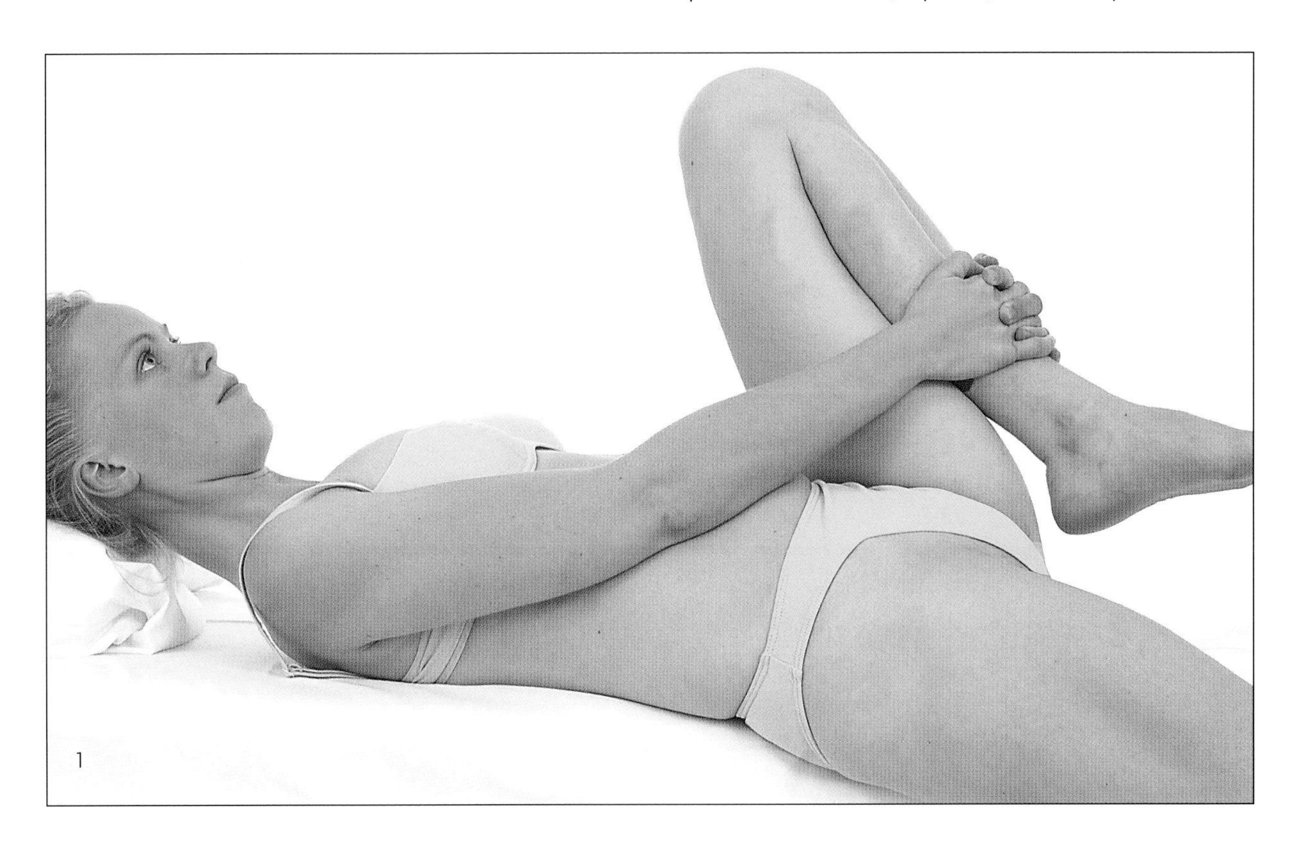
1

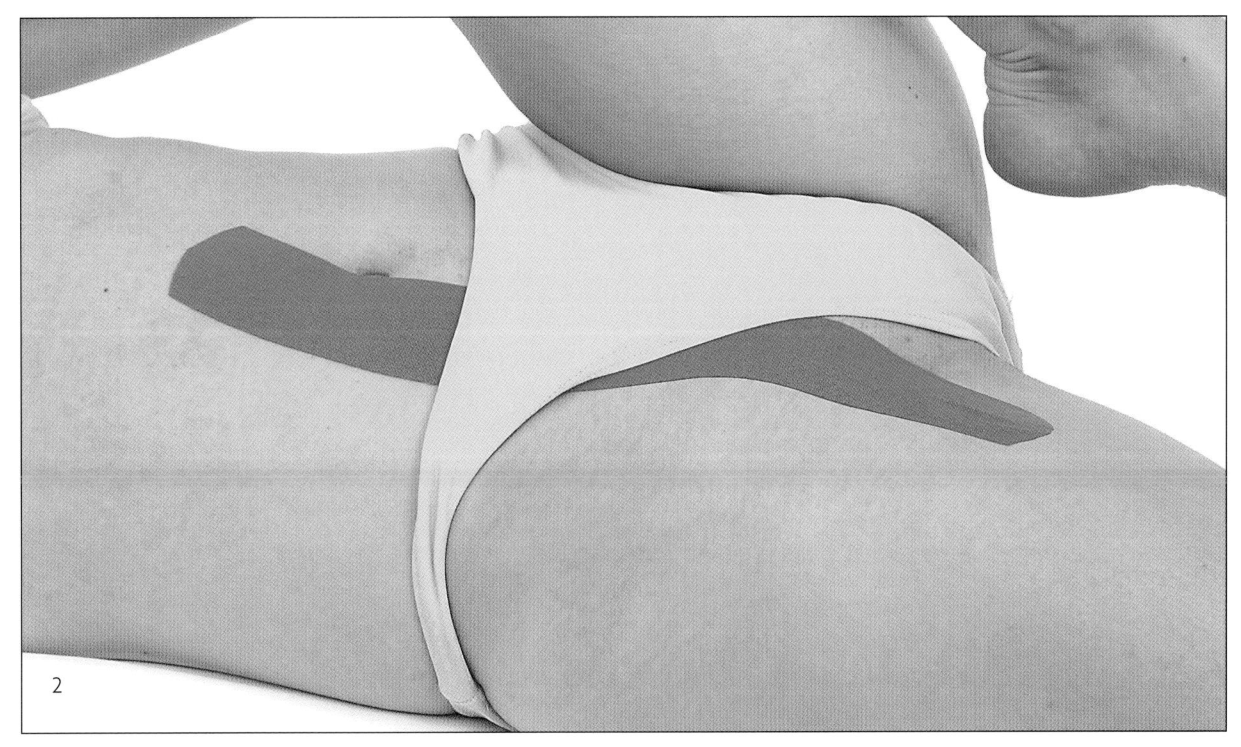
2

22. Knee Tape

Ailments

- Pain in the area of the knee joint
- Knee joint bruise
- Inflammation of the bursa (a fluid-filled sac between a tendon and a bone) in the knee
- Pain in the legs
- Restless legs syndrome

Number and Length of Tapes

Number of Tapes: 2

Measuring the Tape

- **First strip of tape:** Runs from the groin to a little below the kneecap (2).
- **Second strip of tape:** Runs from slightly below the kneecap to slightly above the kneecap (5).

Important: Both strips of tape are cut down the middle far enough that the cut ends can be attached around each side of the kneecap.

Tip: Do a preliminary stretching of the muscles and joints so you can measure the length of the tape strips exactly.

Preliminary Stretching and Attachment of the Tape

Preliminary Stretching

- Recline on a table so that the leg on the side being taped bends at the knee and hangs down over the edge of the table. Bend the other leg so that you can put your foot up on the table (1).

Attaching the Tape

- Set the first strip of tape on the thigh so that the cut end hangs down over the knee (2). Attach the tape from the top of the knee up to the groin (3). Stretch both cut strips of tape slightly and attach them to the right and left sides of the kneecap (3).

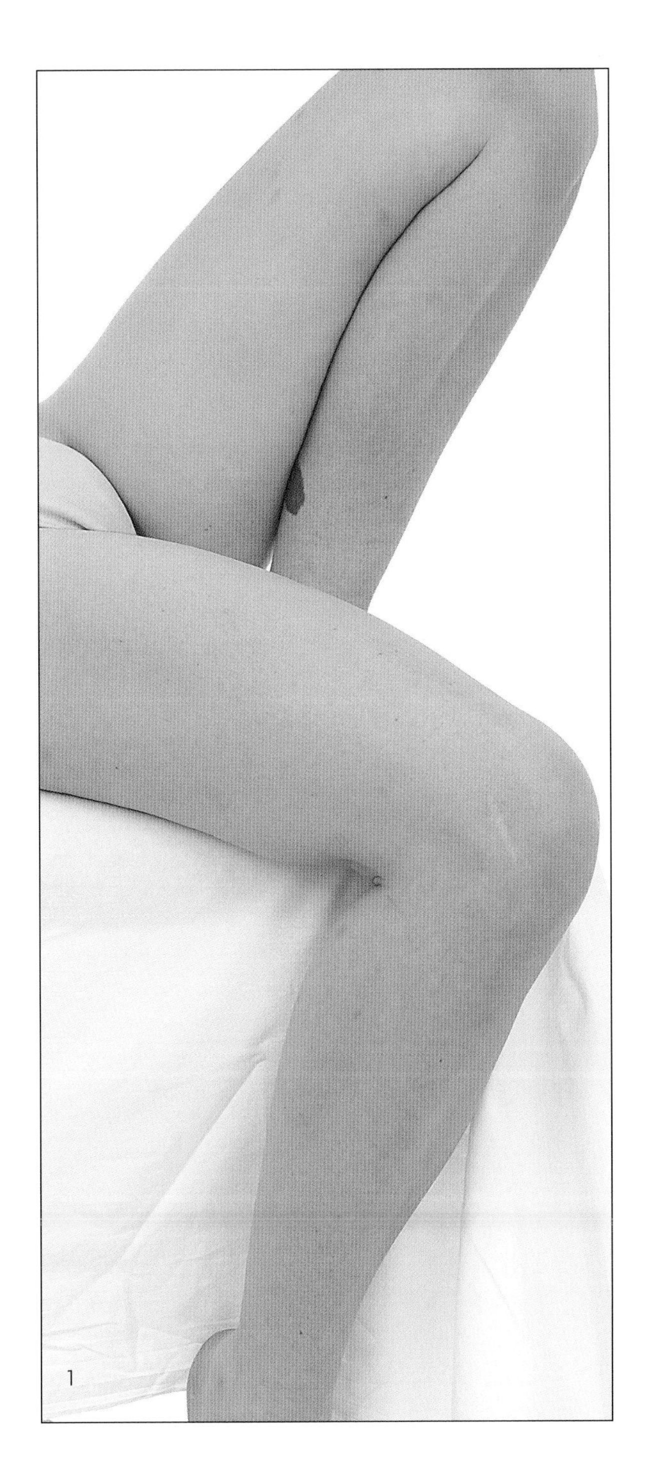

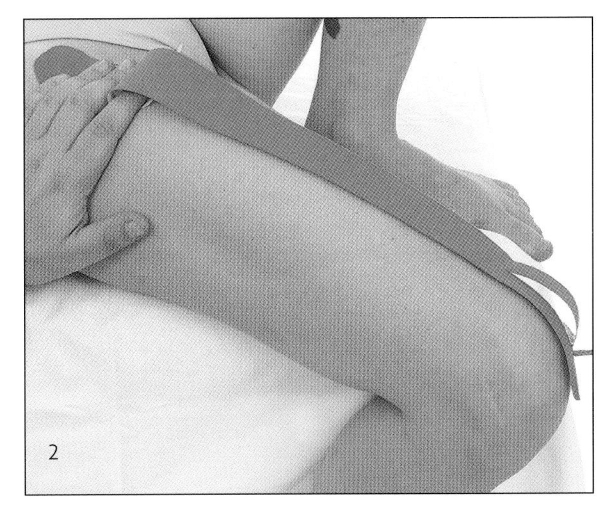

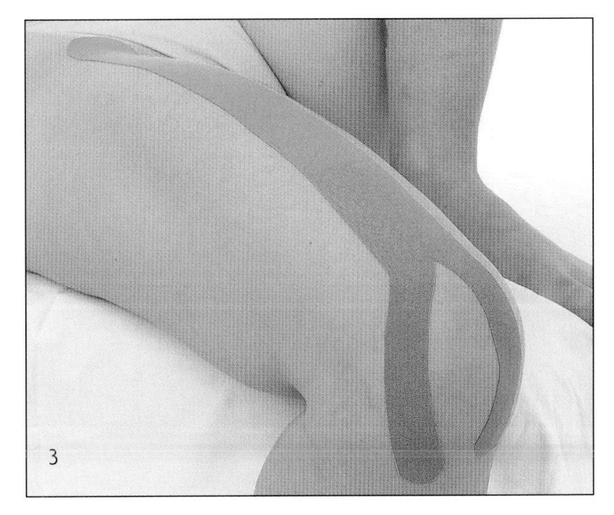

- Attach the uncut end of the second strip of tape along the top of the shinbone below the kneecap so that the cut ends run upward (4). Stretch the cut ends slightly and attach them around the right and left sides of the kneecap (5).

Please Note

- Instead of doing the preliminary stretching as it is described here, you can place a knee roll (a rolled up bath towel works well) underneath the hollow of the knee to create an effective preliminary stretch.
- Two uncut strips of tape can substitute for the second strip of cut knee tape. They can be attached on the right and the left sides of the knee joint as described above (6).

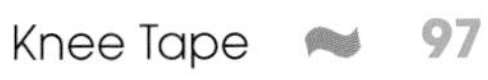

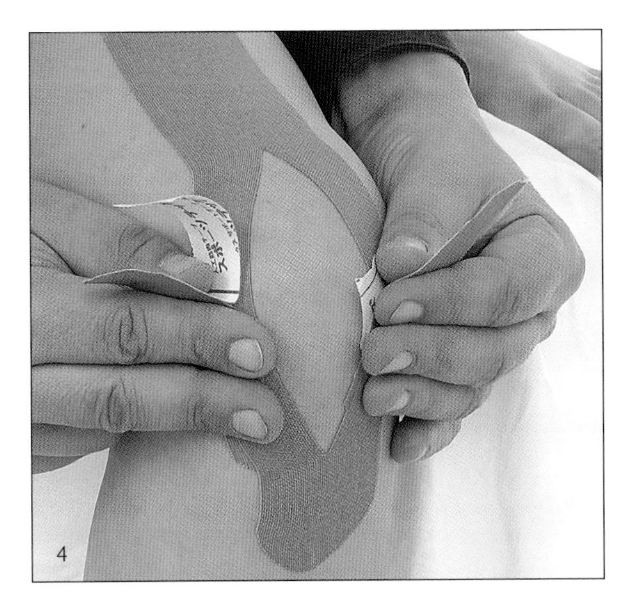

4

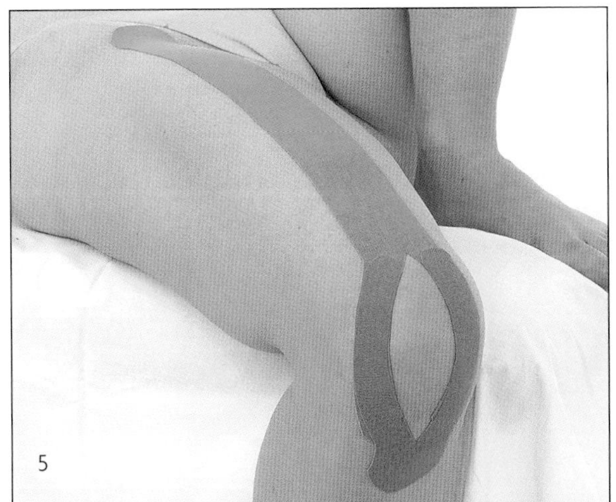

5

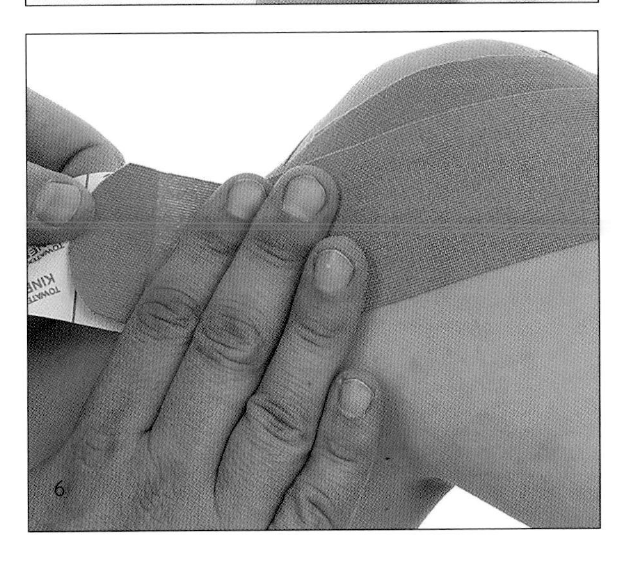

6

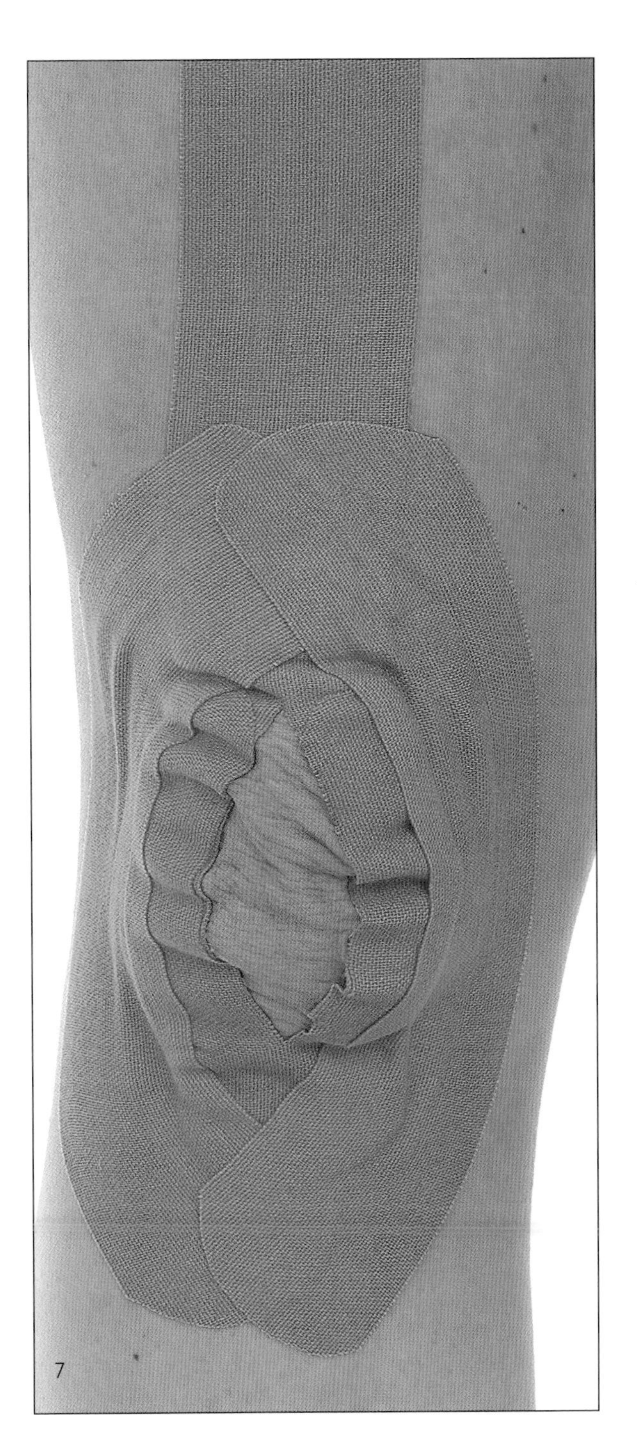

7

23. Combination Tape

Also called pes anserinus (knee joint) tape. For the sartorius muscle, hip joint abductor muscle, and the flexor muscle on the inner side of the knee joint.

Ailments

- Pain in the knee
- Pain in the hip
- Pain in the area of the thigh

Number and Length of Tapes

Number of Tapes: 3

Measuring the Tape

- **First strip of tape:** Runs from the inner side of the knee joint up to the front edge of the hipbone (1).
- **Second strip of tape:** Runs from the inner side of the knee joint up to the crotch (2).
- **Third strip of tape:** Runs from the inner side of the knee joint up to the back of the thigh to below the buttocks (4).

Tip: Do a preliminary stretching of the muscles and joints so you can measure the length of the tape strips exactly.

Preliminary Stretching and Attachment of the Tape

First Strip of Tape

- **Preliminary stretching:** Recline on your back with your legs spread apart as far as possible and stretch the leg that is being taped as far as possible away from you (1).
- **Attaching the tape:** Attach the first strip of tape from the inner side of the knee joint up to the front edge of the hipbone (1).

Second Strip of Tape

- **Preliminary stretching:** Move the leg to be taped a little to the side.
- **Attaching the tape:** Attach the strip of tape from the inner side of the knee joint up to the crotch (2).

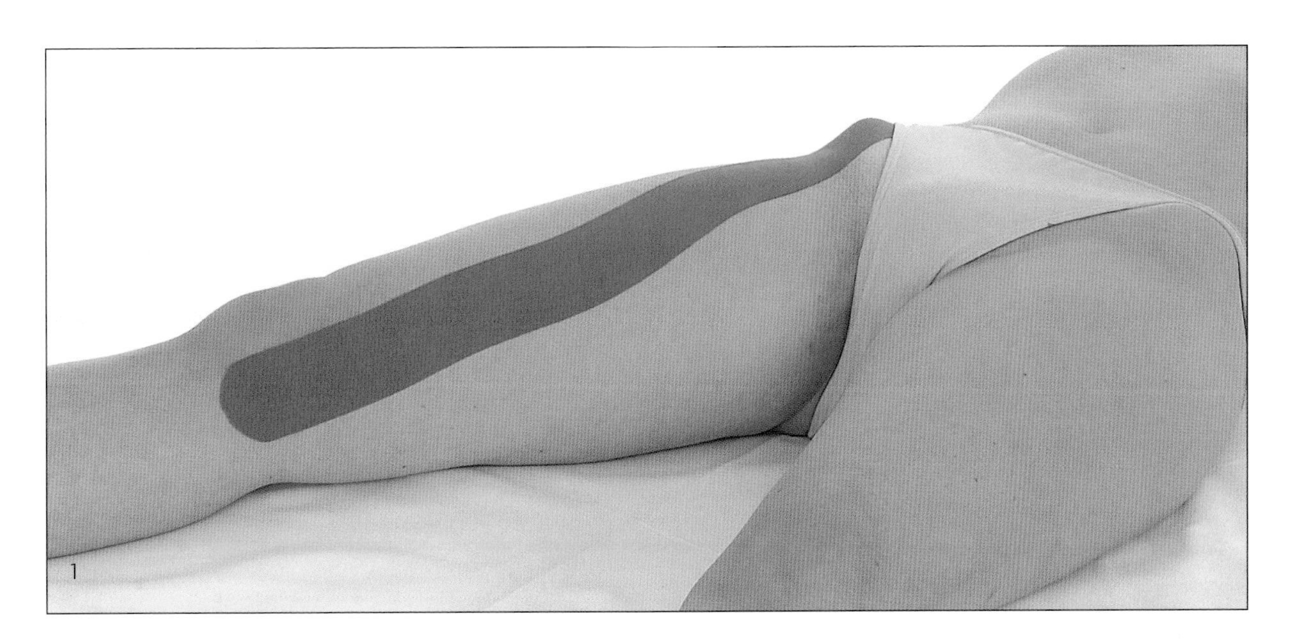

1

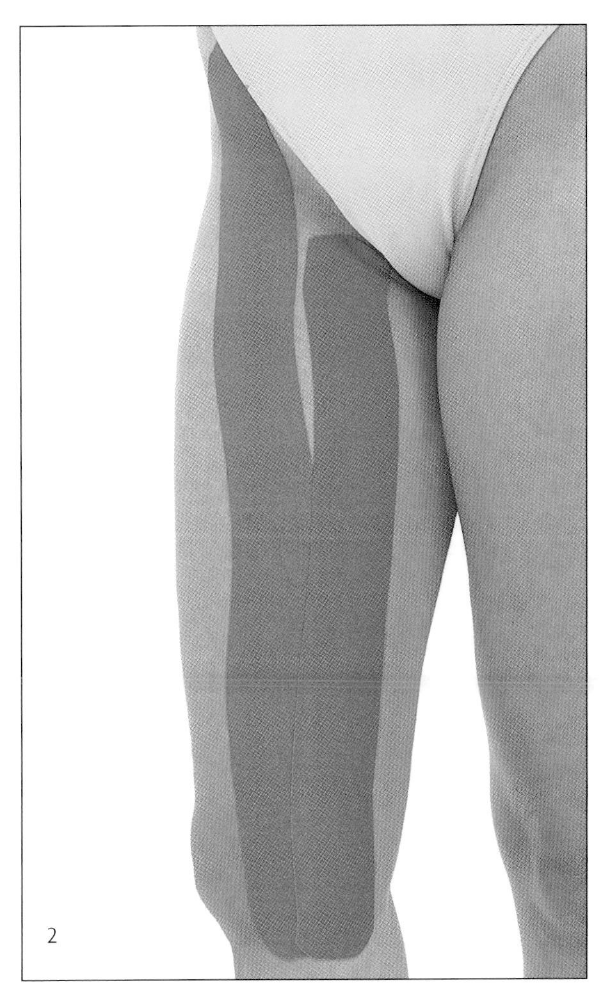

2

Third Strip of Tape

- **Preliminary stretching:** With the taped leg kept straight, pull it up and toward your body with both hands (3).
- **Attaching the tape:** Attach the strip of tape on the inner side of the knee joint up to the ischium (4). The ischium is the lower back part of the hipbone. The ischial tuberosities, sometimes referred to as the "sitz bones," are the part of the ischium that is designed to provide a stable platform when we sit. They can easily be felt in the middle of the lower fold of the buttocks.

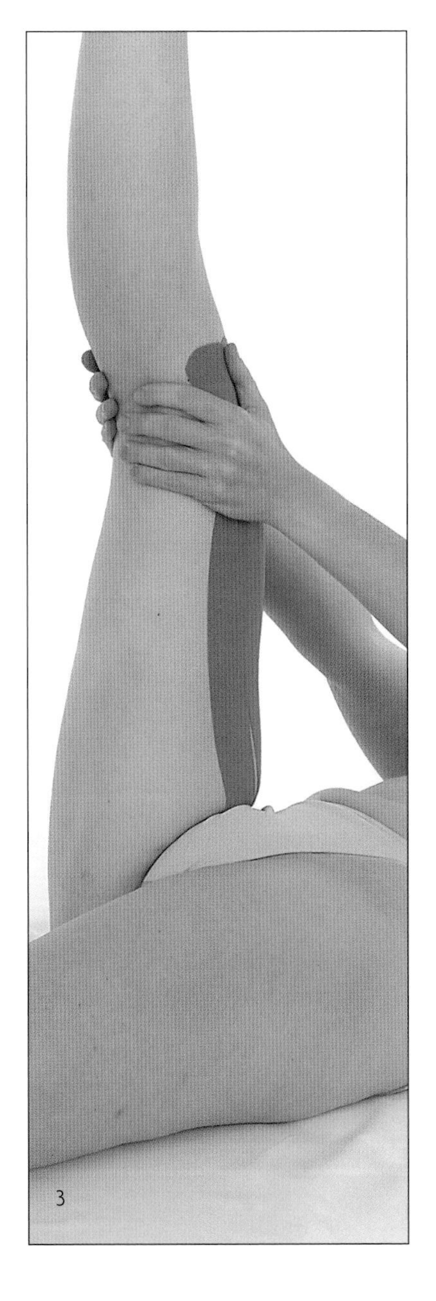
3

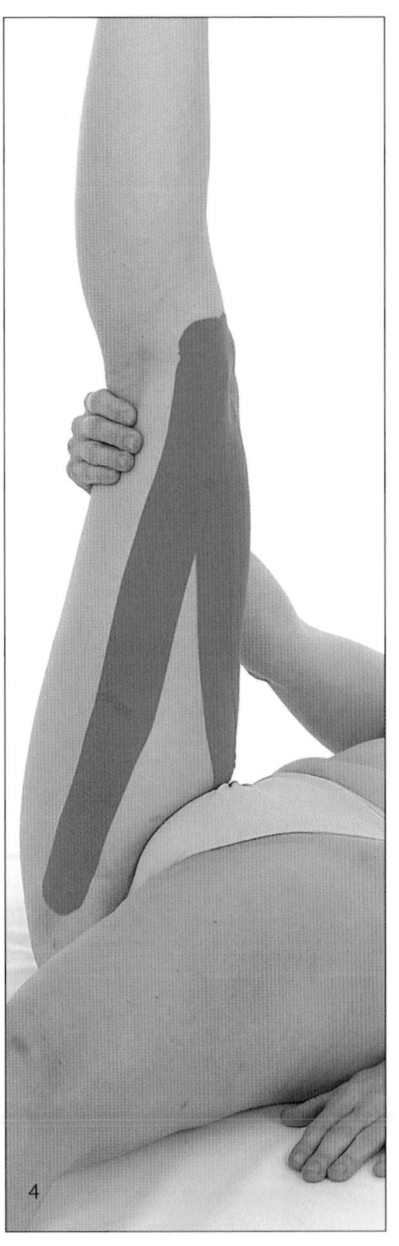
4

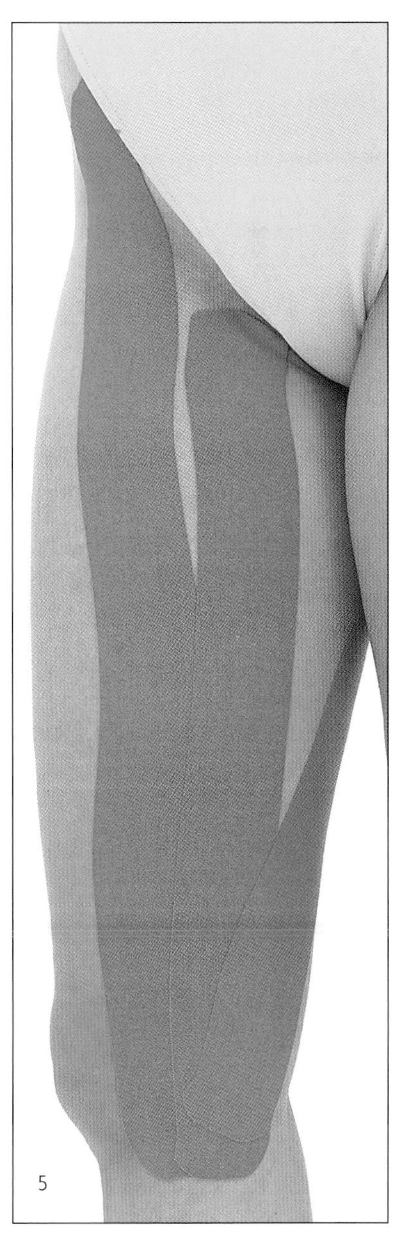
5

24. Knee Flexor Tape

Ailments

- Pain in the hip
- Pain in the area of the thigh

Number and Length of Tapes

Number of Tapes: 2

Measuring the Tape

- Both tape strips run at a slight angle from just below either side of the knee joint to the middle of the lower backside (2).

Tip: Do a preliminary stretching of the muscles and joints so you can measure the length of the tape strips exactly.

Preliminary Stretching and Attachment of the Tape

Preliminary Stretching

- Stand up straight, cross your legs, and bend the upper part of your body forward (1) and down (2).

Attaching the Tape

- Attach the first strip of tape at a slight angle to the left from the middle of the lower backside, over the thigh, to the left side of the knee joint (2).
- Attach the second strip at a slight angle to the right from the middle of the lower backside, over the thigh, to the right side of the knee joint (2).

Please Note

- Because the preliminary stretching should only be done to the best of your ability, it is not absolutely necessary that you cross your legs in the preliminary stretching. Instead, you can stand with them next to each other and just bend the upper part of the body as far forward as possible.
- In medical terminology, this tape also is called an ischiocrural tape.

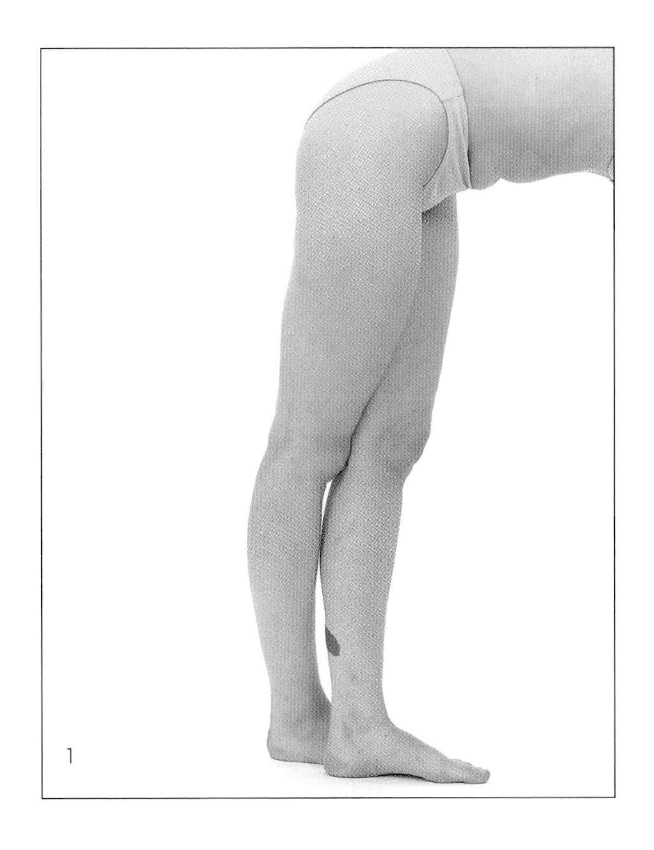

1

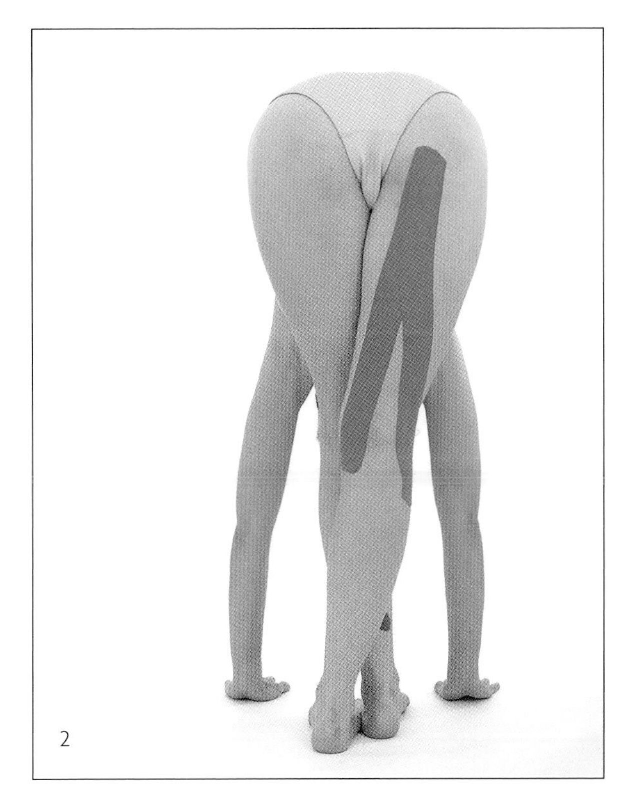

2

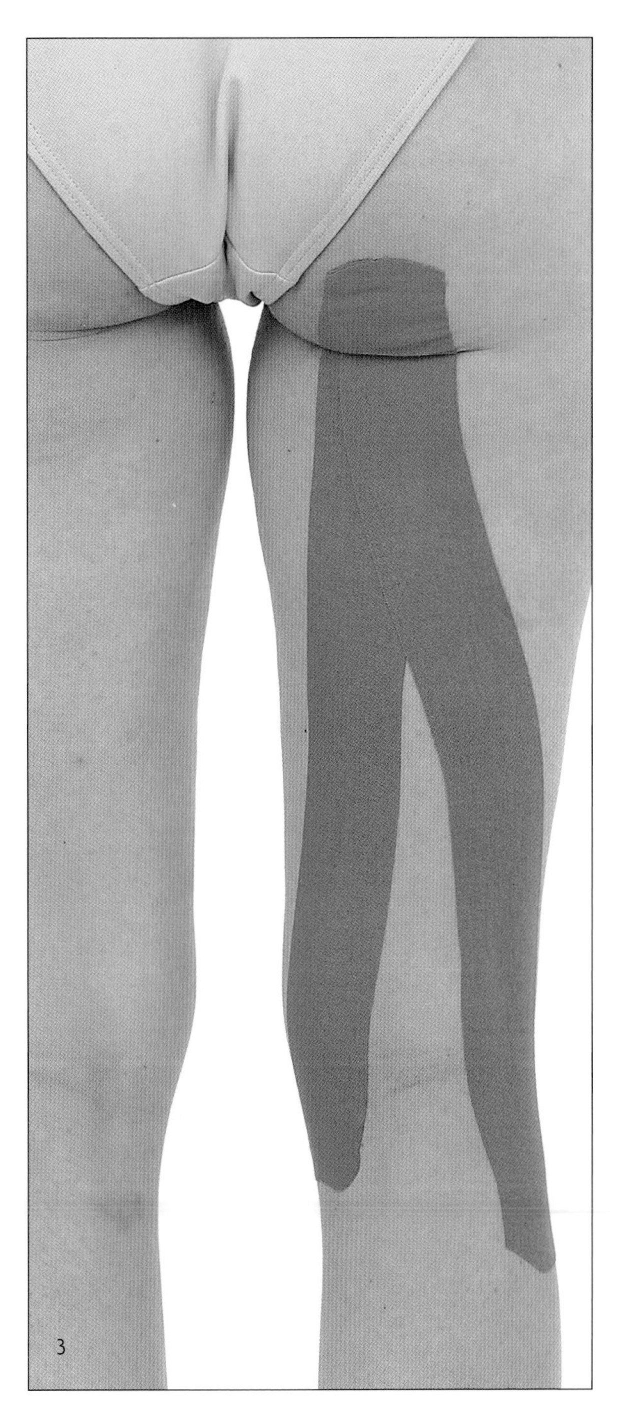

3

25. Achilles Tendon and Ankle Joint Tape

Ailments

- Pain in the leg
- Pain in the Achilles tendon
- Pain in the ankle joint
- Pain in the area of the foot
- Calcaneal spur (spur of the heel bone)
- Cramps in the calf muscles
- Restless legs syndrome

Number and Length of Tapes

Number of Tapes: 3

Measuring the Tape

- **First strip of tape:** Runs from the middle of the sole of the foot, over the heel, up to the hollow of the knee (2).

Important: The tape has to be cut down the middle far enough so that it can be attached in two strips running to the right and the left sides along the calf muscle (2).

- **Second strip of tape:** Runs from the middle of the heel, up the right and left sides of the foot, to the inner and outer sides of the ankle (3).
- **Third strip of tape:** Runs horizontally across the Achilles tendon and over the inner and outer sides of the ankle (4).

Tip: Do a preliminary stretching of the muscles and joints so you can measure the length of the tape strips exactly.

Preliminary Stretching and Attachment of the Tape

Preliminary Stretching

- Recline on your stomach so that a third of the lower leg being taped protrudes over the edge of the bed. Extend your leg and flex the foot so that the toes point up toward the body (1).

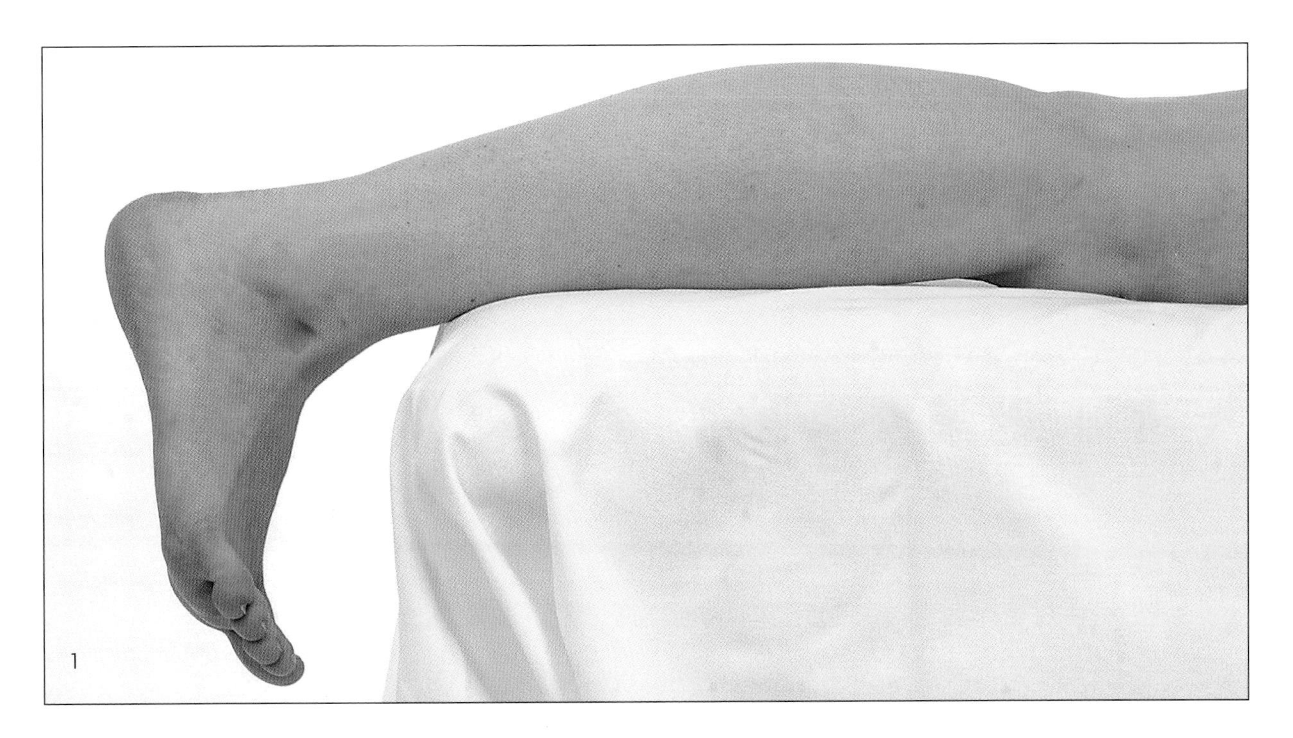

1

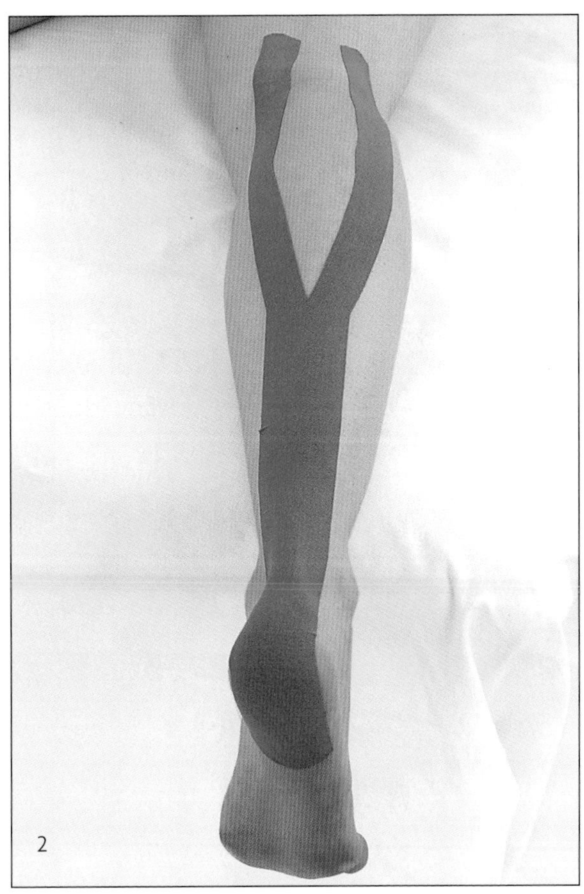

2

Attaching the Tape

- Attach the first strip of tape, starting with the uncut end, from the middle of the sole of the foot up to the beginning of the calf. Then attach the cut ends to the right and the left sides of the calf muscle, up to the hollow of the knee (2).
- Attach the second strip of tape from the middle of the heel to the right and left sides of the foot, up over both sides of the ankle (3).
- Attach the third strip of tape to the right and left from the middle of the Achilles tendon, covering both sides of the ankle (4).

Please Note

- Because it makes sense to use both tapes at the same time, the Achilles tendon and ankle joint tape combines the two taping protocols.

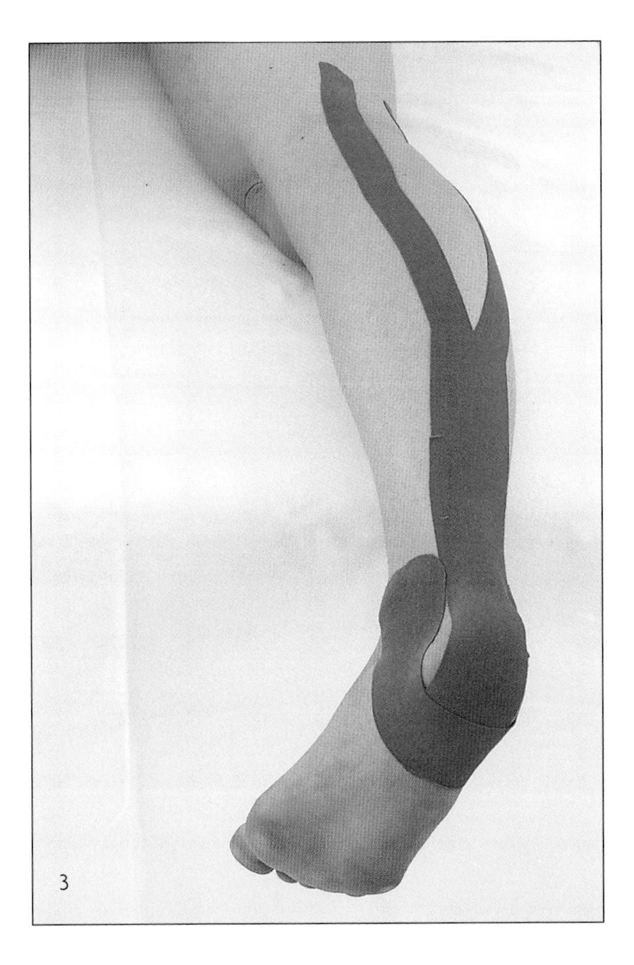

3

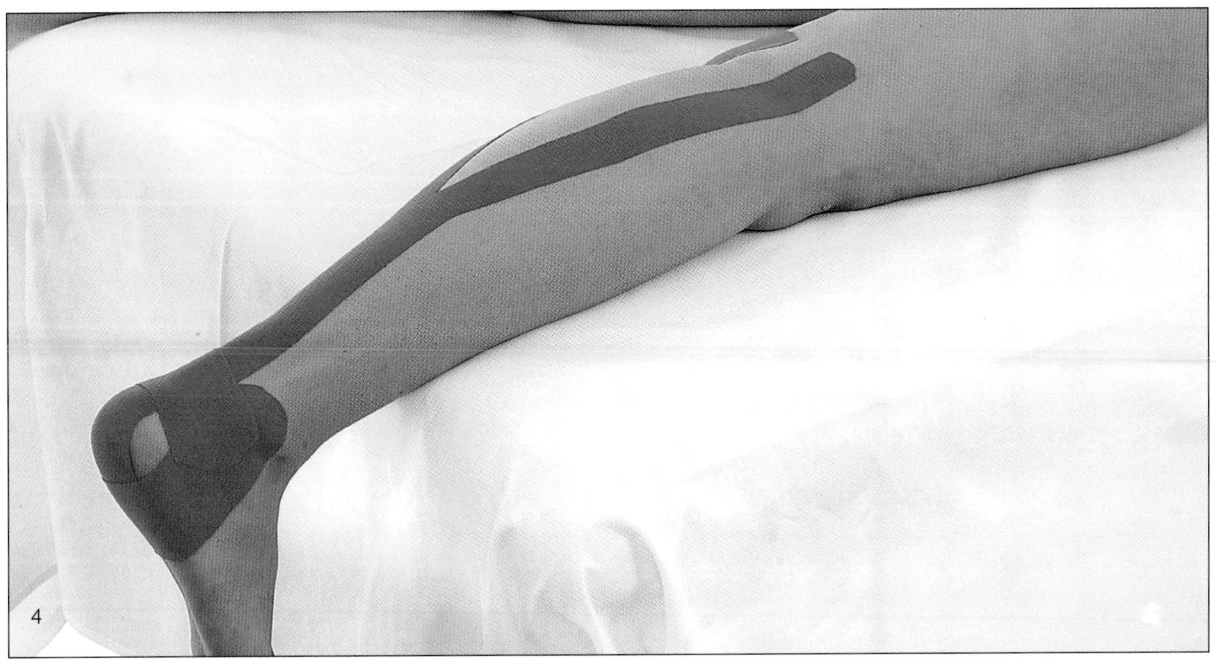

4

Appendix: Ailments From A to Z

In Part 2 of the book, we listed the ailments that can be treated using each particular acutaping protocol. Here you can find all the ailments listed in alphabetical order, the taping recommended for their treatment, and the pages where these treatments are discussed. You will also find those disorders, such as cellulitis and bruising, that were discussed in the first part of the book but do not appear in the practical part for the reason that there are no specific taping protocols recommended for those disorders. Instead, the tape is simply attached over the affected area of the body.

Abdominal pain: Abdominal muscle tape (rectus abdominus), 86–87; abdominal muscle tape (oblique muscles), 88–89; lumbar spine tape, 76–77

Achilles tendon pain: Achilles tendon and ankle joint tape, 104–107

Ankle joint pain: Achilles tendon and ankle joint tape, 104–107

Arm, upper arm pain: Elbow joint flexor tape, 52–53; rotator cuff muscle tape, 62–63; levator costarum (or scalenus) muscle tape, 64–65

Back Pain

Upper back/cervical spine:

- In general: Elbow joint extensor tape, 50–51
- Pain caused by bending and stretching of the cervical spine: Cervical spine tape, 68–71; cervical spine lymph tape, 72–73
- Pain in the side of the body: Cervical spine tape, 68–71; cervical spine lymph tape, 72–73; levator scapula muscle tape, 60–61
- Pain while turning your head: Levator scapula muscle tape, 60–61; levator costarum (or scalenus) muscle tape, 64–65; trapezius muscle tape, 56–59

Middle back/thoracic spine:

- Elbow joint extensor tape, 50–51; thoracic spine tape, 74–75; rhomboid muscle tape, 66–67; pelvic bone muscle tape, 90–91; hip and loin flexor (iliopsoas) muscle tape, 92–93

Lower back/lumbar spine:

- In general: Elbow joint extensor tape, 50–51; lumbar spine tape, 76–77; sacroiliac joint tape, 82–85; pelvic bone muscle tape, 90–91; hip and loin flexor (iliopsoas) muscle tape, 92–93
- After surgery on spinal disc: Lumbar spine tape, 76–77; lumbar spine star tape, 78–81
- Pain that spreads to the outer side of the hip: Lumbar spine tape, 76–77; lumbar spine

star tape, 78–81; sacroiliac joint tape, 82–85; pelvic bone muscle tape, 90–91; hip and loin flexor (iliopsoas) muscle tape, 92–93

Belly area pain: See "Abdominal pain"

Bladder, irritation of: Abdominal muscle tape (rectus abdominus), 86–87; abdominal muscle tape (oblique muscles), 88–89; lumbar spine tape, 76–77; sacroiliac joint tape, 82–85

Bruising: Acutaping of the affected zone, following the direction of the muscle beneath

Calcaneal spur pain: Achilles tendon and ankle joint tape (104–107), attaching from the Achilles tendon to the middle of the sole of the foot

Calf, cramps in the: Achilles tendon and ankle joint tape (104–107), with an additional tape attached, after a preliminary stretching, across the calf

Carpal tunnel syndrome: Finger and forearm extensor tape, 44–45; finger and forearm flexor tape, 46–47; thumb saddle joint tape, 48–49; cervical spine tape, 68–71

Cellulitis: Acutape the disturbed areas of the skin with tape that has been stretched as far as possible before attaching; change tape frequently, every two days or so.

Coccyx pain: Lumbar spine tape, 76–77; sacroiliac joint tape, 82–85; pelvic bone muscle tape, 90–91. As a support, a tape can be attached, after a preliminary stretching, over the tailbone as far down as possible into the fold between the buttocks.

Connective tissue disorder: See "Cellulitis"

Constipation (chronic): Abdominal muscle tape (rectus abdominus), 86–87; abdominal muscle tape (oblique muscles), 88–89; lumbar spine tape, 76–77

Diarrhea: Abdominal muscle tape (rectus abdominus), 86–87; abdominal muscle tape (oblique muscles), 88–89; lumbar spine tape, 76–77

Digestive disorders: Lumbar spine tape, 76–77; abdominal muscle tape (rectus abdominus), 86–87; abdominal muscle tape (oblique muscles), 88–89

Dizziness: Cervical spine tape, 68–71; cervical spine lymph tape, 72–73; levator scapula muscle tape, 60–61; trapezius muscle tape, 56–59; sacroiliac joint tape, 82–85

Elbow pain:

- In general: Finger and forearm extensor tape, 44–45; finger and forearm flexor tape, 46–47; elbow joint extensor tape, 50–51
- Pain that originates in the cervical spine: Cervical spine tape, 68–71; elbow joint flexor tape, 52–53

Foot pain: Achilles tendon and ankle joint tape, 104–107; lumbar spine tape, 76–77

Golfer's elbow: Finger and forearm flexor tape,

46–47; elbow joint extensor tape, 50–51; cervical spine tape, 68–71

Hand, numbness in: See "Carpal tunnel syndrome"

Hand pain:
- Joint pain in the hand: Thumb saddle joint tape, 48–49; cervical spine tape, 68–71
- Pain in the hand on the side of the flexor: Finger and forearm flexor tape, 46–47
- Pain in the hand on the side of the extensor: Finger and forearm extensor tape, 44–45

Hay fever: Cervical spine lymph tape, 72–73

Headaches

Migraine headaches: Acutaping is not an effective therapy for migraine headaches.

Tension headaches: Depending on the location of the pain, different tapes are used.
- Headaches that run from the back of the head to the front or the eyes: Cervical spine tape (68–71) in combination with the cervical spine lymph tape (72–73) and the levator scapula muscle tape (60–61)
- Headaches in the temples: Cervical spine tape (68–71) in combination with the upper and middle strips of the trapezius muscle tape (56–59)
- Headaches in the front of the head: Levator costarum (or scalenus) tape, 64–65; cervical spine tape, 68–71
- Headaches originating in a functional disturbance of the cranial joints and the sacroiliac joint: Sacroiliac joint tape, 82–85

Hip pain:
- Originating from the lumbar spine: Lumbar spine tape, 76–77; pelvic bone muscle tape, 90–91; sacroiliac joint tape, 82–85; hip and loin flexor (iliopsoas) tape, 92–93
- Pain in the area of the upper forward edge of the hipbone: Combination tape (pes anserinus tape), 98–101
- Pain in the area of the back of the hip running into the hollow of the knee: Knee flexor tape, 102–103

Incontinence: Abdominal muscle tape (rectus abdominus), 86–87; abdominal muscle tape (oblique muscles), 88–89; lumbar spine tape, 76–77

Joint, bruises of: See "Joint pain"

Joint pain: Acutaping of the affected joint. In addition, other tapes can be attached at the side of the joint.

Knee pain:
- In general: Combination tape (pes anserinus tape), 98–101
- Pain on the inner side: Knee tape (94–97) with an enhancement on the inner side
- Pain on the outer side: Knee tape (94–97) with an enhancement on the outer side
- Inflammation of the bursa (a fluid-filled sac between a tendon and a bone): Knee tape, 94–97

Knee joint, bruise in the: Knee tape (94–97) with several amplifications on the inner side and outer side

Legs:

- Restless legs syndrome: Knee tape, 94–97; lumbar spine tape, 76–77; Achilles tendon and ankle joint tape, 104–107
- Pain in the leg: Pelvic bone muscle tape, 90–91; knee tape, 94–97; hip and loin flexor (iliopsoas) tape, 92–93; lumbar spine tape, 76–77; Achilles tendon and ankle joint tape, 104–107
- Pain in the area of the thigh: Knee flexor tape, 102–103; combination tape (pes anserinus tape), 98–101

Menstrual pain: Sacroiliac joint tape, 82–85; lumbar spine tape, 76–77; lumbar spine star tape, 78–81; abdominal muscle tape (rectus abdominus), 86–87; abdominal muscle tape (oblique muscles), 88–89

Muscles, pulled: Acutaping of the pulled muscle area and the neighboring joints

Muscles, sore: Acutaping of the affected zone and the neighboring joints

Neck pain: See "Back pain" and the "upper back/cervical spine" listing

Pregnancy, pain during:

- Pain in the abdominal area: Abdominal muscle tape (rectus abdominus), 86–87; abdominal muscle tape (oblique muscles), 88–89; lumbar spine tape, 76–77
- Pain in the area of the back: Lumbar spine tape, 76–77
- Pain in the lower back that spreads to the thoracic spine area: Lumbar spine tape, 76–77; thoracic spine tape, 74–75; possibly sacroiliac joint tape, 82–85
- Vomiting (nausea) during pregnancy: Finger and forearm flexor tape, 46–47

Rib cage pain: Pectoral muscle tape, 54–55; thoracic spine tape, 74–75

Ringing in the ears: Cervical spine tape, 68–71; levator scapula muscle tape, 60–61; trapezius muscle tape, 56–59; sacroiliac joint tape, 82–85; cervical spine lymph tape, 72–73

Scars, clearing the effect of (interference suppression): Acutaping of the scar. The tape should be stretched as far as possible before you attach it and it should be changed frequently—every two days or so.

Shoulder pain:

- In general: Trapezius muscle tape, 56–59
- Depending on the main pain area, two tapes maximum: Levator scapula muscle tape, 60–61; rotator cuff muscle tape, 62–63; pectoral muscle tape, 54–55; elbow joint extensor tape, 50–51; elbow joint flexor tape, 52–53; levator costarum (or scalenus) tape, 64–65; rhomboid muscle tape, 66–67

Sinusitis: Cervical spine lymph tape, 72–73

Tailbone pain: See "Coccyx pain"

Tendonitis (inflammation of a tendon): Finger and forearm flexor tape, 46–47; thumb saddle joint tape, 48–49

Tendosynovitis (inflammation of the fluid-filled sheath surrounding a tendon): Finger and forearm extensor tape, 44–45; finger and forearm flexor tape, 46–47; thumb saddle joint tape, 48–49

Tennis elbow: Cervical spine tape, 68–71; finger and forearm extensor tape, 44–45; finger and forearm flexor tape, 46–47; elbow joint extensor tape, 50–51; elbow joint flexor tape, 52–53

Thumb, pain in the area of the base of the thumb joint: Thumb saddle joint tape, 48–49

Tinnitus: See "Ringing in the ears"

Afterword

The acutaping therapy presented in this book can be very beneficial in the treatment and healing of disorders. We believe that with this form of therapy we can give patients with chronic pain the opportunity to undergo an effective treatment procedure and at the same time enable them to actually be directly engaged in the process themselves, actively participating in the work of their own therapy. It is this active engagement in the therapeutic work of treating one's own ailment that we feel can be the first step in a successful outcome. It is always important, though, that your complaints be checked out beforehand by a doctor.

With this in mind, we wish you the sensible dash of sceptical objectivity that can keep you from making mistaken assumptions and misinterpretations that can come as a result of the sometimes spectacular successes of acutaping.

At the same time we do wish you all the success in the world with this unique treatment—of course!

Sources of Acutape

Acutape is readily available online and over the phone under the name *kinesio tape*. It is sold in the United States, Canada, and internationally. A single 4.5-yard roll of tape goes for anywhere from $12 to $16 per roll. Most suppliers also sell boxes of two, four, or six rolls of tape or longer bulk rolls at lower prices per foot.

You are not likely to find the tape in your local drugstore. A medical supply store in your area might carry it, or be able to order it for you, but in our experience it's not always possible to buy single rolls of tape through your local store.

We have listed several sources below, which will provide easy access to the tape in a variety of colors, widths, and lengths.

Informational Web Sites

Both of these sites also sell kinesio tape online or over the phone at the numbers listed.

Kinesio Taping Association
www.kinesiotaping.com
Kinesio USA, LLC
3939 San Pedro Drive NE
Albuquerque, NM 87110
Phone: 888-320-TAPE [8273]
or 505-856-2029
Fax: 505-856-2983
E-mail (for information):
info@kinesiotaping.com
E-mail (to order products):
kinesiousa@kinesiotaping.com
This site lists a number of U.S. distributors of Kinesio Tape. It also lists international sources for the tape, including distributors in Japan, Korea, the United Kingdom, Germany, Belgium, Italy, and Spain.

Kinesio Taping in Canada
www.kinesiotape.ca
Dr. Roger Berton (contact person)
1041 Lesperance Rd.
Tecumseh, Ontario
N89 1W9
Canada
Phone: 519-979-2663
Fax: 519-979-2286
E-mail: drrogerb@yahoo.ca

Other Sources for Purchasing Tape

OrthoCo, Inc.
www.orthoco.com
P.O. Box 208
Cherry Hill, NJ 08003
Phone: 856-795-6900
Fax: 856-795-6922
E-mail: sales@orthoco.com

OrthoCanada
www.orthocanada.com
OrthoCanada Medical Products
37 Katimavik Road
Val-des-Monts, QC
J8N 5E1
Canada
Phone: 1-800-561-0310
Fax: 1-800-561-0349

Amazon.com
www.amazon.com
Just type in Kinesio Tape for product options.

The Supply Stores
www.medsupplystore.com
Jerabek & Co. DBA The Supply Stores
1424 4th Street Suite 212
Santa Monica, CA 90410
Phone: 800-441-2850
Fax: 310-362-8648
A user-friendly site that is a particularly good source of individual roles of tape at reasonable prices.

Index

Please note that numbers in *italics* indicate illustrations

About the Authors

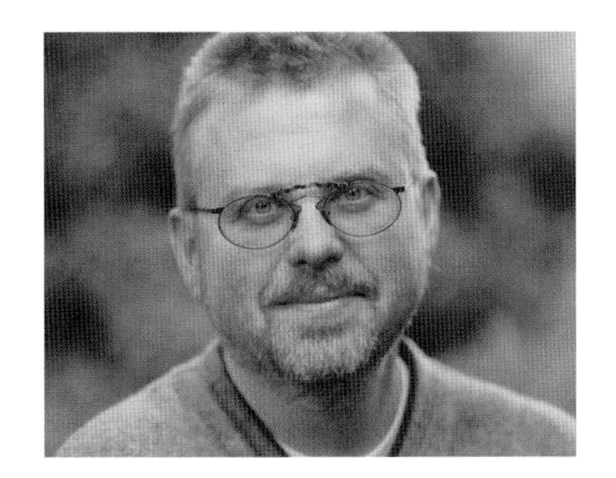

Hans-Ulrich Hecker, M.D., is an internationally known expert in acupuncture and Chinese medicine. In his numerous publications (translated into many languages), Dr. Hecker helped make traditional Chinese medicine popular and helped to establish the acceptance of its methods for use alongside conventional medical practice in the doctor's office. Since 1990, he has been a medical specialist in general practice, homeopathy, naturopathic treatment, acupuncture, and medical quality management, and he shares his knowledge with interested colleagues. This "master of the delicate pinpricks" is the head of advanced training for acupuncture and naturopathic treatment of the Medical Association of Schleswig-Holstein. Since 1993, he has held a position as a lecturer for acupuncture and naturopathic treatment at the University Clinic, Schleswig-Holstein Campus in Kiel, Germany. Together with Dr. Kay Liebchen, he developed acutaping.

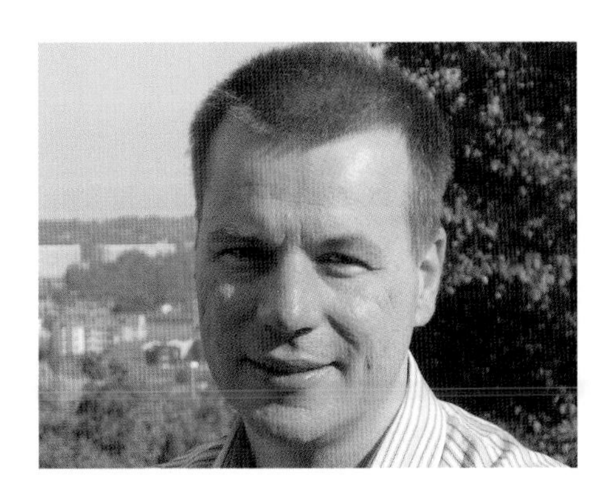

Kay Liebchen, M.D., is a registered orthopedist in Schleswig, Germany, with an emphasis on rheumatology, special pain therapy, acupuncture, osteopathy, and acutaping. From 1997 to 2004, he was head of the department in the pain clinic at Damp, Germany, and helped with its setup. He has been teaching chiropractic techniques since 1995 at the Dr. Karl Sell Medical Seminar, which is held at the training facility in Damp. As a lecturer on acupuncture at the training academy of the Medical Association of Schleswig-Holstein, his emphasis lies in the combination of acupuncture with manual therapy and osteopathy, trigger point therapy, and acutaping. Dr. Liebchen is also co-author of a number of books.

BOOKS OF RELATED INTEREST

Trigger Point Therapy for Myofascial Pain
The Practice of Informed Touch
by Donna Finando, L.Ac., L.M.T., and Steven Finando, Ph.D., L.Ac.

Trigger Point Self-Care Manual
For Pain-Free Movement
by Donna Finando, L.Ac., L.M.T.

The Encyclopedia of Healing Points
The Home Guide to Acupoint Treatment
by Roger Dalet, M.D.

The Acupressure Atlas
by Bernard C. Kolster, M.D., and Astrid Waskowiak, M.D.

The Reflexology Atlas
by Bernard C. Kolster, M.D., and Astrid Waskowiak, M.D.

The New Rules of Posture
How to Sit, Stand, and Move in the Modern World
by Mary Bond

The Reflexology Manual
An Easy-to-Use Illustrated Guide to
the Healing Zones of the Hands and Feet
by Pauline Wills

Reflex Zone Therapy of the Feet
A Comprehensive Guide for Health Professionals
by Hanne Marquardt